Women in therapy and counselling

Women in therapy and counselling

Out of the shadows

Moira Walker

Open University Press
Milton Keynes · Philadelphia

Open University Press
Celtic Court
22 Ballmoor
Buckingham
MK18 1XW

and
1900 Frost Road, Suite 101
Bristol, PA 19007, USA

First Published 1990
Reprinted 1992
Copyright © The Author 1990

British Library Cataloguing in Publication Data

Walker, Moira
    Women in therapy and counselling.
    1. Women.   Psychotherapy
    I. Title
    616.8914088042

    ISBN 0 335 09376 0
          0 335 09375 2 (pbk)

Library of Congress Cataloging-in-Publication Data

Walker, Moira, 1948–
    Women in therapy and counselling: out of the shadows/Moira
    Walker.
        p.   cm.
    ISBN 0-335-09376-0.   ISBN 0-335-09375-2 (pbk.)
    1. Women—Mental health.   2. Women—Social conditions.
    3. Women—Counselling of.   4. Psychotherapy.   I. Title.
    RC451.4.W6W35   1990
    362.83—dc20   89-78214 CIP

Typeset by Gilbert Composing Services
Printed and bound in Great Britain by
Woolnough Bookbinding Limited,
Irthlingborough, Northamptonshire

For Tessa and Sarah with love and hope

Contents

Preface and acknowledgements

This book has arisen from many years of working in Britain with women as a social worker, teacher and trainer, and as a counsellor and psychotherapist. Although written primarily from that standpoint, my own experiences of being a woman will also have influenced its writing. Although I remain amazed at the burdens of suffering and abuse so many women carry, I also recognize the resources women have within them. Most cope and survive. Many do so extraordinarily well, going from strength to strength. For others it is more marginal. A few have not survived, and I carry the memory of those few with me.

In many ways writing this book is a tribute to women in their various struggles. It could not have been written without all those I have worked with in various capacities. I would like to thank them: I have gained from working and being with them. Sharing and knowing their struggles has at times given me needed strength. I hope this book will be of interest both to men and to women, but in particular to the large numbers of people in a variety of settings who work so hard to care for women, often with little support or recognition, and with few resources. Many women will recognize aspects of their own lives in these pages; perhaps they will draw comfort from knowing that they are not alone.

As the reader will see, considerable use has been made of case material, and indeed the first two chapters are based on this. Great care has been taken to preserve confidentiality. In fact, although the originator of 'Suzanne' was happy for her case history to be used, she would not now recognize herself. While preserving the basic structure of family patterns, other radical changes have been made. This is true of all the case material used. Throughout, the terms 'counselling' and 'psychotherapy' have been used interchangeably. This has been intentional, but does not imply that I see no distinction between the two. I believe there are differences, but this is not the place to debate the point. The issues discussed in these chapters relate to both, wherever the line is drawn between them.

Writing this book has both delighted me and daunted me. As always, the support and interest of many people have been sustaining and stimulating. Too many of my friends and colleagues have contributed, knowingly or not, for me to thank them all individually. But I do thank them all. Some special thanks are due: to my friend and colleague, Michael Jacobs, for his ongoing support and encouragement; to my daughters for their interest, tea and sympathy, and tolerance (and occasional intolerance, reminding me firmly of worlds beyond the word processor); and to my friends, Inge and Malcolm Roberts, for friendship and support over many years, and in many ways. Thanks are also due to my sister, Gillian McCredie, for her considerable help in providing information and material, especially for Chapter 7. Barbara Webster and David Brandon have made helpful comments on different chapters at different times, and their encouragement has been much valued.

1

Suzanne's story

The box is locked, it is dangerous.
I have to live with it overnight
And I can't keep away from it.
There are no windows, so I can't see what is in there.
There is only a little grid, no exit.

Sylvia Plath

For the counsellor the arrival of a new client is an everyday and familiar occurrence. For the client it is not. For her it is a unique experience – one that brings with it a mixture of feelings – anxieties, fears and hopes. To talk to a stranger suggests that other routes have not worked, that they have been insufficient, or that they have not been appropriate. It may be felt that friends, partners or relatives are unable to cope with the contents of that 'box' to which Sylvia Plath refers – that what it contains may indeed be too dangerous, too destructive and too powerful; that the risk of revelation is too great to take. It may also be that those very people who it is generally assumed will be there to give support and care are themselves part of the difficulty; and, of course, for some women that network of support may simply not exist.

When a new client asks for therapy or counselling she will be aware that all is not well in her world. Sometimes the cause of this feeling will to some extent be clear – it may be an immediate but unmanageable response to a tangible and obvious event or problem; or it may appear to be such, yet also carry with it unresolved traumas from the past that are triggered by recent real events. Often it will be a feeling of great distress which is overwhelming, but which is not obviously explicable, which feels impossible to resolve and is an alarming scenario to explore alone. Yet, unexplored, it becomes more dangerous. The contents of the locked box, while unfamiliar, are open to distortion, realities becoming indistinguishable from fantasies. What belongs to the past and what, correctly, needs seeing as the present, is no longer clear. It becomes difficult to know which strands are really significant, and which are not.

As a result, a newly arrived client is likely to feel, to put it simply, in a muddle. She will often have no idea where to begin, which strand to select, or if indeed it is safe to select any. There will be many questions in her mind. What will this person she has come to see be like? Will s/he listen, understand, take her seriously? Will s/he pass judgement on her; maintain confidentiality; like her; and be able and willing to help? Some clients, in their unhappiness and distress, very much want their counsellor to 'make them better'; and most counsellors, when faced with such distress, would dearly love to be able to do so. But magic wands do not exist, and an approach is needed that takes careful and real account of these complexities, and actively acknowledges both the present and the past as always having significance for women.

The present and the past cannot be seen as existing in purely individual terms. They must, to have validity and meaning, also be seen in the context of a wider society, and of the culture, history and politics of that society. If proper attention is not given to this wider picture, then the view of women, and the view for women, will inevitably be distorted. Significant and often powerful forces will be ignored. It is equally important, however, that the similarly powerful forces of individual development and dynamics are given adequate acknowledgement; otherwise, in a parallel manner, the picture will become equally distorted.

Clearly the various aspects of women's lives do not fall neatly into tidy categories; rather there is an ebb and flow between them. There are no neat lines in the lives of people, but there are forces, demands and injunctions that come from inside and from outside the individual. Where, and at which point, the outside forces meet the inside forces, and vice versa, and whether this distinction is ever constant or always moving, is obviously a question for ongoing debate. But at least awareness of the question identifies the existence of the issues, and hopefully prevents simplistic assessments from being made. Assessments of women in the past have too often been made in the context of a society that has been (and still is) male-dominated, and that has often seemed unable, or unwilling, or both, to look at the resulting difficulties for women.

The presenting problem

In many ways, and at many levels, the story of Suzanne, as it unfolded over a period of eighteen months in therapy, illustrates these points. Hers was not in itself an unusual situation to bring to therapy – a feeling of quite severe depression that she herself was unable to make sense of. Her story has a particular value and uniqueness, in that, as it unfolded, so did the stories of her mother and her grandmother before her. In total this represented a hundred years in the lives of three women in one family, covering a period of time that encompassed two world wars, the introduction of the welfare state, and a myriad of legislative, social and political changes. Within this history lay patterns of living and being that emerged, which finally enabled Suzanne (once they had been painfully disentangled) to progress in her own life and in her own way, with more belief in herself.

Suzanne, in the telling of her story, took her time. In the first few weeks of therapy an outline of herself and her life began to emerge, and as time went by more of the pieces began to fit together. It was immediately apparent that she was experiencing quite severe depression, that this was very frightening, that she could not understand it, and that the suicidal feelings that accompanied her depression were very alarming to her. She was very tearful and distressed. Until recently she had been a part-time teacher, and was now undertaking further studies to improve her qualifications. It was at the start of these studies (she was a mature student among a much younger age group) that she suddenly began to feel very depressed. She had looked forward to resuming her studies, and could think of no reason why she should be feeling this way.

Early weeks in therapy

As the first few weeks passed, more detail of her life and history emerged, particularly relating to her husband and children. Her husband was a successful accountant. They had met at college when they were both nineteen. They had married on completion of their studies, and he now had a well-paid and prestigious job, involving considerable travel away from home. They had two daughters, aged eleven and sixteen, who appeared to present no particular difficulties. Suzanne had been depressed on several occasions in the past, although never, she felt, as seriously as at present. Her first memory of depression was of episodes during her college days, although she could not explain these. Following the birth of her first child her depression had returned, and had been severe enough for her to be prescribed anti-depressants. She was again depressed when her first child was four, although on that occasion she managed without anti-depressants; but they were prescribed again when her second child was five.

Suzanne was herself confused by this history of depression. She could not make sense of it, nor did she understand what had triggered these feelings; she only knew that after a while they had gone away. Now she was feeling very bleak again; all around her seemed black, at a time when she felt everything should be feeling good. After all, she told herself, she had financial security, two nice children, a husband, and a career which she was beginning to develop further. Why, then, was she feeling so bad, so bad that on some days she felt she did not wish to carry on?

At this stage she did not say much about her relationship with her husband except that they got on well. Although he did not know just how bad she was feeling at present, he was genuinely concerned. Yet as he was very busy at the moment she did not want to pressurise him any further. She felt he had been supportive in the past, for instance when she had gone back to work after the birth of their first child. At that time she had given up her job, due to her anxieties about the care of the baby, but her husband had tried to reassure her: he had felt the baby was fine with her childminder, yet was also concerned that Suzanne should not feel pressurized to work if she was not happy to do so.

Her wider family history was at this time also alluded to, albeit briefly. Her mother was still alive, and they 'got on well'. She had one younger sister. Her father had died some years previously. She had coped with his death well, unlike her mother and sister, who had been 'very distressed'. It also transpired that although Suzanne felt she had some good friends, they were geographically scattered. There was no one living nearby in whom she could confide. The people she knew locally 'just wouldn't understand'. It was evident that she was feeling very lonely and isolated.

The significance of the early weeks

As always, the initial stages of contact between client and counsellor are significant and full of meaning for both of them. Some of the client's initial questions will have been answered, although others will remain, while still more are likely to lie dormant, unexpressed as yet and often at this stage unrecognized. But at least the unknown person in whom Suzanne, in her great unhappiness, had chosen to confide was now becoming more familiar. She had the security of knowing that she would be seen regularly, at a given time, for a specific length of time each week. At this point in the relationship with her therapist, Suzanne was beginning, tentatively, to feel a little safer, and knew she would be listened to and taken seriously. This in itself should never be underestimated as being helpful in its own right, although, as we shall see, this was not in itself going to be sufficient for her. But at this stage Suzanne herself was able to express clearly the value she placed upon their meetings:

> It's really mattered that you've listened to me, and taken me seriously. It's felt like a huge weight lifted off me. When I have bad days I try and tell myself to hold on, and that I'll be able to tell you about it.

This feeling of relief is, of course, frequently expressed by women who have so often carried a real burden of responsibilities: for their children, for their partners, for their jobs, for their homes, and for others – for some women the list is endless. To an objective outsider it may seem amazing that they have coped so well with so much for so long, but many women will often not share this perception of themselves and will feel they are not coping. This is perhaps because so many of women's responsibilities are relatively invisible, and are not given much credence or value by our wider society. Until, that is, something goes wrong, such as in childrearing, when women all too often take the blame. The converse is not true: that is, women are rarely given the credit when all goes well. It certainly seems exceedingly difficult for many women to acknowledge their own strengths, perhaps because they have so soaked up the popular mythology of men being strong and women being weak.

As we can see with Suzanne, the very fact that she was listened to, taken notice of, and taken seriously, gave her at this early stage a little relief from her loneliness and despair. As we shall see later, these early and positive feelings towards her therapist developed as time went on, and began to allow room for some rather more negative ones, too. These more negative feelings, allowing free expression within a safe relationship, were central to the understanding of Suzanne's difficulties.

The early sessions clearly had considerable impact upon Suzanne, but it is also important to look at the significance of the first few sessions for Suzanne's therapist. What was she thinking during this time? How did she share this with the client? She felt that she was beginning to make sense, for herself and for Suzanne, of what was certainly experienced by her client as a frightening and quite severe depression. Some of this understanding is described below.

However, it is important to recognize that there is always a danger in a counsellor or therapist jumping to conclusions too quickly about what may or may not be 'the problem'. Such conclusions are even more dangerous if they are reached and acted upon unilaterally, without checking out their validity with the client. Favourite ideas and theories, books recently read and too rapidly digested, or the latest conferences attended, should be seen as valuable extensions to a tenative knowledge base, but not as newly discovered panaceas.

Too rapid and too definite a conclusion can be unhelpful in other respects, too. Once a problem has been defined in a certain way, it can thereafter be difficult to 'undefine', particularly if such a definition is a safe, acceptable and comfortable one for both client and counsellor. Women coming for therapy or counselling often feel in their distress that they would just like the therapist to take all their troubles and pain away. This is not in itself an unreasonable feeling. What is unreasonable is for the therapist or counsellor to collude with this expectation, because this is again to reinforce the experience, often described by women, of someone with 'expert' knowledge 'knowing' what the problem is, and even defining it in stereotypical terms such as 'just their time of life', or 'the time of the month', or 'women are over-emotional', as though the cause were obvious and simple, and the solution known. Such a response increases the power differential between therapist and client, when, more appropriately, efforts need to be made to minimize it.

Using Sylvia Plath's vivid image of 'the locked box', too early and precise a description of the contents can make further exploration of other parts of the box very difficult. It may well be true that its top layer can be described accurately, but what may actually be needed is to look beneath what is immediately visible. In order to do this both client and therapist need to work, as far as possible, as equal partners.

Exploring possible pathways

The problems of making early and rigid diagnoses can best be illustrated by examining more closely the material which Suzanne herself provided in those early sessions; by explaining how her therapist understood what she was being told; and by considering the implications such thinking could have for a possible 'treatment plan'. Different initial assessments obviously carry with them the possibility of distinct paths of exploration for the client. Some pathways can be too rigidly mapped before the journey of exploration starts, allowing no chance for deviation. Others permit time and space to pause and reconsider as the journey progresses. What possibilities and pathways might be considered to be available to Suzanne and her therapist?

If the therapist feels that no significance should be attached to the past, the aim of the exercise being simply to rid the client of troublesome symptoms, s/he is likely to see any previous history of depression as irrelevant to the present symptom. Instead, s/he may feel that it is entirely appropriate to work in a defined and short-term manner with a particular focus on certain aspects of the client's life. In this case, therefore, s/he will concentrate on Suzanne's thought and/or behaviour patterns.

Alternatively, it can be argued that Suzanne is entering a period of 'mid-life crisis' where many real life changes are indeed taking place. She appears socially isolated, her children are growing up, she has entered a new and strange world, and it is possible that she is not getting much support from her husband. With such understanding as a basis for counselling, it might be appropriate to occupy a supportive role for Suzanne while she passes through this transitional phase of her life; and it could be helpful to suggest joining a women's group, both in terms of consciousness-raising, and for further support for her.

Another approach is to define Suzanne's situation as a marital problem, and her depression as an expression of unhappiness and anger with her husband, both for being too busy to recognize how depressed she is, and for building and developing a successful career and somehow leaving her behind. In this instance marital therapy may be seen as potentially most effective.

Others may see Suzanne's depression as chemically caused, and not as a reaction to events or circumstances. In this case referral to a doctor might be suggested, remembering that Suzanne had been prescribed anti-depressants on previous occasions, and so may herself see these as helpful.

However, there are two questions to be asked at this point. First, do any of these explanations really touch the level of depression which Suzanne is experiencing? Second, if a woman's history is to be seen as having any significance, do any of these explanations help us to understand the pattern of depression over the years? These are questions which a therapist is likely to ask, although not solely of herself: they can be explored with the client, to find out whether or not these possibilities may be relevant.

Let us check through the various explanations outlined above in relation to Suzanne's story and to what she was saying about herself. Suzanne was adamant that she did not wish to take anti-depressants again – she did not wish to be 'all fogged up', as she put it. The possibility of looking at her relationship with her husband was also inappropriate at this stage, because she was not able to look at this area of her life. It did not feel safe for her, and this was acknowledged by both therapist and client: they agreed to look at the relationship as and when Suzanne felt it appropriate.

It could be argued that her reluctance to talk about her marriage indicated that this was problematic, but it was also clear that to have time that was hers and hers alone, neither shared with nor invaded by anyone else, was something which Suzanne valued enormously. To have taken that away from her and put her in the arena of joint marital therapy when she was both vulnerable and saying she did not want it, could be seen as anti-therapeutic. She was able, however, to acknowledge that she did find it difficult to know what she could reasonably expect from her husband. She could not tell where legitimate requests and expectations ended nor what were unreasonable demands.

She was able to recognize that she had the same difficulties in friendships; and, very hesitantly, she began to experience the same uncertainties and anxieties in relation to wanting more from her therapist. She began to acknowledge that she found it difficult to trust people, which left her quite bereft and alone at times. It was significant for both Suzanne and her therapist that at an early stage this aspect was identified and agreed upon as a problem area. Similarly, it was important that Suzanne was able to see that she was anxious about her children starting to grow up. Although this was initially expressed as concern for their well-being, she saw that a more important question was whether she could cope with the separations and transitions which their growing up would inevitably involve. A much fuller understanding of this aspect of Suzanne's difficulties emerged as time elapsed, but the early identification and sharing of this were important, even at such an early stage.

What, then, was the picture which the therapist was left with after these few early sessions? Inevitably, of course, the picture was still very fuzzy. Some shapes were emerging, but they were lacking in form and content; they were vague outlines rather than definite objects. Some dimensions of the picture were looked at by Suzanne and her therapist together, including those already described above. But other questions and thoughts remained in the therapist's mind, although at this stage they were kept to herself as matters for her own thinking and perusal. There is always a dilemma over the timing of interventions. On the one hand, the therapist wishes to share thoughts and ideas as honestly as the client is encouraged to. On the other, the client needs to proceed at her own pace, unpressurized by the therapist's thoughts, which may in any case not always be entirely relevant to what the client feels at any particular point of time. It should be said that the conflict between wishing to give space, and the wish to share honestly, is not peculiar to the therapeutic relationship; it can exist between any two people who are close. There is no clear answer to this dilemma, although a useful guideline is to explore and suggest tentatively, while always giving the client the opportunity to reject, accept, or defer as she sees fit.

The thoughts in the therapist's mind at this early stage were various. One area of thinking that she was able to share usefully with Suzanne was that her current life experiences and situation did not seem to explain sufficiently either her present level or her past history of depression. In other words, while acknowledging her present realities, and the problematic nature of some of these, as well as actively acknowledging the distress and fear caused by the depression, there remained an overall question of the fundamental nature of Suzanne's difficulties. Was there a pattern to these recurring episodes of deeper unhappiness, and, if so, could unravelling the pattern help prevent its continuation? The therapist was also asking herself questions about the significance of the death of Suzanne's father, with which, in her own words, she had 'coped well'. She was wondering what this really meant, and about her overall relationship with him. Gentle hints in this direction were firmly rejected by Suzanne: it felt very much a 'no-go' area, in much the same way as her relationship with her husband was similarly not allowed on the agenda at this time.

While the therapist in no way wished to pressurize Suzanne into areas she did not want to explore or did not feel were relevant, it was nevertheless important to be able to put to her that these were two people, so significant in her life, whom she found it hard to talk about. It was also put to her cautiously that it may have been hard for her to express her needs to either of them, and that she may have been left with angry feelings about this, which were also difficult to express. It was carefully suggested that it might be hard, too, for her to tell her therapist what she wanted, or what she felt in the therapeutic relationship, particularly where this involved negative feelings. Suzanne was certainly able to identify with this, and was relieved that it could be expressed and recognized by someone else. The recognition that her depression was not a simple response to a given incident or situation, but that it was deeper and more complex than this, made her feel less alone in her unhappiness. She was not only concerned to make sense of this, but also very frightened at the prospect of doing it. To put it in her own words: 'I don't know if I'm going to find nasty skeletons in the cupboard; and if I do, if I'll be able to cope with them.'

Acknowledging such fears and ambivalence is always an important part of therapy and counselling. It is perhaps also important to offer some reassurance: if skeletons do appear they can at least be examined together; and, generally speaking, a visible skeleton is preferable to an invisible ghost. It is then identifiable, and its reality becomes available for inspection. This can be painful, but there is a sense of moving forward, rather than living with the fears and fantasies of what the skeleton may really look like, or what damage it may do.

It was at this point in therapy that Suzanne and her therapist agreed to continue to work together on an open-ended contract, that is, without yet setting a definite finishing date. It was perhaps because of this that space was given for a much fuller picture of her life to emerge.

Suzanne's developing relationships

In many ways Suzanne's early history will be very familiar to those families who faced the separations engendered by the Second World War. Suzanne was born in wartime. Consequently, she had practically no contact with her father as a small child. He was on active service and she had no early memories of him, except as a vague and shadowy figure who would occasionally appear only to disappear again. However, she did not remember these as unhappy years. Her maternal grandmother lived with her and her mother. Suzanne was devoted to her, and felt they were a very happy trio. How much of this was an idealized picture, particularly in terms of her later experiences, was hard to tell, but it certainly appeared that Suzanne had received some good early care and nurturing.

When she was two years old her mother returned to work, part of the body of women who, at a time of labour shortage, became a sought-after resource for wartime production. Suddenly, it appeared, women were able to do jobs previously denied to them; suddenly it was deemed that it was not necessarily harmful for small children to be left in the care of others. Such is the nature of political expediency! While her mother worked, Suzanne was cared for by her grandmother. She did not feel this was anything other than a good time in her life. Her grandmother liked caring for her, her mother liked working; and apart from occasional and (she remembered) rather confusing and unsettling visits by her father, she felt she was a secure and at that time a happy child. She remembered her father's visits being anticipated as special times, and how she had felt (as she could now define it as an adult) that somehow the expectation and the reality did not quite match up. This experience had caused her some unexpressed anxiety even as a child. She had always known that she was supposed to be excited by the arrival of this special person, but somehow it had not quite felt like that, and his arrival felt more like the invasion of a stranger.

The age of five was in many ways a watershed for her. She started school; her father returned home; her mother, like many women of the time, reluctantly gave up her job; and her grandmother moved out of the family home to live nearby. This was not a happy time for the family: Suzanne felt ill at ease with her father and missed her grandmother; her mother missed her job. A year later, when Suzanne was six, her sister was born; the baby was adored by her father. Suzanne remembered feeling lonely and isolated, and spending much of her time with her grandmother, who was in considerable conflict with her father. At school she succeeded academically, and made some friends, but she was very much seen as a quiet child. At the age of eleven the family moved house, and Suzanne changed schools. She was very unhappy at this time: she did not like her new school, and missed her regular contact with her grandmother. When she was thirteen she was moved to a boarding school. Fortunately it was a caring school, and she settled well, but she had not been there long when her grandmother died. She did not attend the funeral, and it was never discussed with her afterwards. She continued to do well academically throughout her school years. She had friends, but none to whom she was very close. After leaving school, she spent a year working abroad, and she remembered this as a happy time in her life.

She met her husband, as already indicated, in the first few weeks of her college life, and they married as soon as they left. She described their relationship as 'companionable' though never passionate, but they lived together amiably enough while he pursued his career in accounting, and she became a teacher. They both worked, bought a house, and were busy improving both their home and their career prospects. When their first child was born - Suzanne was in her late twenties, and at that time her husband's career was at 'take-off point'. She was a happy, easy baby, but Suzanne became depressed and anxious, although her husband, when he was at home, was supportive and involved with the baby. Suzanne attempted to return to work, but felt unable to continue, and did not return until both her children were of school age. Between the birth of her two children she was never really happy, but she felt better after the birth of her second daughter, although she was a difficult and restless baby. At this time her husband changed his job and was at home more. She again had periods of depression when each of her children started school, but these gradually lifted and the period of part-time work before she started her studies seemed a time of some equilibrium for her.

Before looking at the specific issues, it is important to understand that such a synopsis of a life story may communicate information, but it gives little else. The printed word cannot adequately convey the quality and depth of the despair and anguish felt by the client, re-experienced in the telling of her story. Often there emerge for the first time parts of the self, and parts of the past, which if not entirely forgotten have been successfully repressed for a long period. Sometimes bits of the story have been told to different people, but because of this have never been joined together. The parts apparently do not belong to each other, and are not always related as aspects of the same experience. Such partial storytelling and remembering is a protection against painful scenarios emerging, but there is always the danger, as patterns become more entrenched, that they become less easy to understand, and, as with Suzanne's depression, are eventually expressed in alarming symptoms. Suzanne had never told any one person all that she had told her therapist. She had told bits to her friends, to her husband, to her children, but in a very matter-of-fact manner, as interesting but not particularly noteworthy. It appeared that no one had ever picked up the discrepancy between the words, so casually expressed, and the meaning, so deeply felt.

Unravelling the issues

A detailed picture of Suzanne's life and experiences has been drawn in order to demonstrate how many dimensions there were to her story. It was this detail that enabled Suzanne and her therapist to begin to unravel some knots and examine more of the strands, and that process will now be described. It will be remembered that areas that had been raised so far related to her relationship with her father and her husband; issues of trust (and the implications of this for the therapeutic relationship), and of concern over making unreasonable demands. There were also issues to do with separations and transitions, although in the early weeks these were not very explicit. As Suzanne's story emerged, so did a pattern in her life. Particularly important was the emerging recognition that some patterns were intricately weaved through the lives of not only Suzanne but also her mother and grandmother.

Issues of loss and separation were of paramount importance to Suzanne, and caused her considerable distress and anger. It has been noted already that these were touched upon in the first few weeks, in relation to children growing up and eventually moving away; but underlying this theme were many unresolved losses and separations belonging to her past. Indeed, simply to have taken the question of growing children at face value would have in all likelihood effectively prevented the further exploration that was to prove so significant.

The feelings connected with separations and losses were extremely frightening for Suzanne. There had been many such times in her life, and those involving her grandmother had lain unexpressed for years. She had never been able to explain to anyone just how important her grandmother had been to her. She had mentioned her death to others, but for most people the death of a grandparent, while being a sad loss, is not a momentous event. Death is expected as old age progresses, and when it comes it may not be a terrible blow. But for the thirteen-year-old Suzanne it was devastating. She did not grieve. She was not comforted. She felt alone with her feelings and confused by them. Her confusion was great because in her eyes she had suffered the most enormous loss, but apparently it was not seen that way by anyone else. She felt as if she had no right to grieve, and that grief was her mother's prerogative. She felt, rightly or wrongly, that any expression of her own needs would be seen at home and at school as making demands she had no right to make. This, of course, repeated the patterns of the earlier situation in relation to her grandmother: when Suzanne was five her grandmother left home to make way for her father, who was a 'returning hero'; her father felt like a stranger and she missed her grandmother, but again in this situation she had been unable to express her feelings. Indeed, as an adult looking back, she felt that her five-year-old intuition was likely to have been correct. It would not have been acceptable to have rejected her father and made a bid for her grandmother. Then she had a further separation from her when she was eleven. Once more her grief and her anger went unexpressed and unseen.

It is possible to understand from all this the intensity of Suzanne's feelings as she uncovered these aspects of her life, and as the pieces of the jigsaw started to fit. The reader, too, may make some sense of the feelings of despair, anger and hopelessness that resulted from the death of someone so close to the young Suzanne. However, when these pieces combined with other, even earlier experiences, the effects were devastating and long-lasting. At the age of five, the person who cared for Suzanne was usurped by a virtual stranger, at least in her own eyes. He was not the stranger who brought happiness and excitement, which had been promised. For her, there was a large gap between the myth of his return, and reality as it was experienced. But the myth meant that Suzanne had no right to complain: she was supposed to be pleased. She was not allowed to say what she wanted, to express how she felt. If she had done so it would somehow have meant that she was 'bad', 'naughty' or 'unreasonable'. We can only guess, too, at the measure of the anger a small child feels when the person s/he loves most is taken away, and how frightening that anger can be when locked inside.

It is also worth observing, as Suzanne came to recognize, that it was a man who returned; it was a man who had the power to do all this to her. Neither she nor her mother or grandmother were able to do anything about it. She was able to make the link herself to her angry, mistrustful and despairing feelings, that men come and go at will (as her husband had done with his job); that they take others away, and that they do not meet or even recognize your needs. For her, men became experienced as very powerful and women as powerless. Associated with all this was a feeling of guilt which had been very deeply repressed, that somehow it had all been her fault, and that the transformation of her life from a happy one to a sad one when her father had returned would not have happened if she had felt the way she 'should' have done. We will see later how this developing picture helped Suzanne and her therapist to understand the pattern of depression in her adult life. There were other key issues which Suzanne came to identify as important. Trust has already been mentioned, and this was present as an issue in the therapeutic relationship as well. This was a huge difficulty for Suzanne. She was quite evidently able to make caring relationships, as long as she was firmly the carer. She certainly gave her own children excellent care, and appeared to be a competent and confident teacher. This was not unexpected in someone who had received loving care herself as a small child. Her problem was receiving care for herself. She could not trust that such care would not be withdrawn, and consequently found it very hard to express the needs she so strongly felt. The resulting combination of anger and loneliness was a powerful one, especially when particular life circumstances meant that her own needs were unusually strong.

This difficulty in trusting was linked to anxiety about closeness and dependency; she saw these as dangerous, although also as needs which she would dearly love to have met, while not believing they ever would be. Her anxiety made life very problematic at those times when dependency was unavoidable. She could not believe, if she allowed herself to trust, or allowed herself to get close, that it would not all be taken away from her. It was safer, on one level at least, not to take that risk. Unfortunately, as she discovered, taking that path had its costs too: it did not relieve past hurts, and the void it left inside her created new agonies.

In addition to all these difficulties, Suzanne was able to express her concern, an overwhelming one at times, about being a 'good mother'. She felt very strongly that 'they mustn't go through what I did'. Inevitably her anxiety and her guilt that she was not fulfilling her own high expectations were at their greatest when she was feeling depressed. This in truth reinforced her fears, at a time when they had some basis in reality. There was a real danger of her creating a self-fulfilling prophecy, that would then precipitate even greater depression, a vicious circle of guilt and despair.

As she expressed these feelings, Suzanne and her therapist began to make sense of the depression which she had initially presented as her main problem; they were able to make links to experiences in the past. Unravelling these was a tortuous process, in which Suzanne came up against pain, anger and distress. But there was some enlightenment and clarity, as she herself became able to see the picture of her life emerge in a much fuller and less shadowy way. Suzanne could see the shadows and confusions which had previously obscured the picture. She recognized how her periods of depression all occurred at times when issues concerning separation and loss came to the fore; or when there were questions about her dependency on others. Sometimes, of course, these coincided.

She could therefore make sense of the times when she became depressed as a young college student at the beginning and end of term. She had not only to separate at these times (from those at home or from her boyfriend at college), but because of her difficulty with this, she was also faced with uncertainties about her dependency needs. She was able to identify how the birth of her first child had brought all these factors powerfully into play. She felt she had lost her previous equal status with her husband; she had lost her career; and the birth itself felt like a separation. But on top of all this the baby was good; and everyone was delighted, making her feel that she should be delighted, too. This last aspect, as she came to realize, was a repetition of her early childhood experience when, as we have seen, she felt she had to behave and respond in one way to her father's return, when she was actually feeling the opposite. When her baby was born, just as when she was five years old, she felt the injunction from others that she should be happy, and that this should be a time for celebration and joy. Negative feelings were not acceptable, and if she expressed them that would make her unacceptable. At five she was trapped in the myth of the returning hero; in her twenties she was trapped by the equally powerful myth of glorious motherhood. Her later feelings were further compounded by her anxieties about dependence at a time when both financially and emotionally she had become dependent. In her own eyes it was as if she had become a child again. She could recognize, too, that when her first child was born, she had to repress all the rage inside her, since this rage made her feel very guilty. She believed that everyone was being 'good' except her. It also seemed that her feelings of guilt and her fears of being 'bad' made it more difficult to return to work, since she had to prove that she was a 'good mother'.

Suzanne was able to see how this pattern continued. For instance, she coped better with her second baby, who was a far more demanding child. In her own words:

> I felt easier with her from the start, and much more in sympathy with her. I think, in a funny sort of way, she was expressing a lot of

the things I couldn't. She could be very demanding at the most inconvenient times. And I can remember not feeling resentful, but thinking 'good for you'. I wish I could have been like that. And, because she was difficult, people didn't expect me to be so happy and cheerful all the time. It was all right to be tired and grumpy.

Two further episodes of depression occurred when each of the children started school. Suzanne again experienced feelings of loss and anxiety, and was eventually able to see that these feelings were only marginally to do with her own children, who apparently separated without difficulty. The experience recreated in her, very powerfully, her own anguish and despair as a five-year-old starting school. Her starting school coincided with her grandmother leaving and her father returning. Of course, at the time, she had not been able to express the grief, anger and fear at having her life so inexplicably disrupted in so many ways at once.

Past history, present feelings

All this helps to explain why the feelings of depression that Suzanne presented to the therapist later in her life could not be explained simply by the circumstances of the present time. Nevertheless, we are still left with an important question: even if the underlying causes were indeed multi-faceted and deeply rooted, what was happening both in Suzanne's external life and in her internal self to act as a trigger for such enormous despair at the time she came for therapy? To understand this trigger, we need to look at how Suzanne viewed the question of her own potential professional success, and her return to study. One part of her knew that she was extremely able and competent, and that she had the ability to do well, possibly very well. Part of her very much wanted this. But she was tremendously ambivalent for many complex reasons.

First, returning to full-time study was a major decision for her. In taking it, she felt she had said goodbye to the part of her life in which she had been, in her own assessment of herself, primarily a mother. Moving away from that felt a huge loss, triggering for the first time her own childhood experiences of loss of mothering. She realized that she had been able to meet some of these mothering needs in herself by appropriately and successfully meeting those of her children. Returning to study meant an acknowledgement that this stage of her relationship with her children would change, as her younger daughter joined the older one in adolescence. This made her very aware of a void within herself.

Second, there were issues involving her husband, reflecting the complex interaction between the history of past dynamics and present-day realities. She was feeling very angry with her husband. Her entry into a younger world, in which she perceived that issues of sexism and inequality were being recognized, actively discussed and encountered, led her to a more active encounter with her own personal situation. She did not like much of what she saw. She began to identify her feeling, which had lain dormant for some time, that her husband's own career success had come about at the expense of her own; and that a relationship which had started off with the promise of equality, had moved a long way from that ideal. Now she felt that his apparent encouragement of her return to study was only superficial, and that his words were not being backed up by actions.

This slotted into Suzanne's history. She was unable to express her anger and resentment directly towards her husband, just as it had been difficult for her either to show negative feelings or to make known her own wishes towards or about her father. This was further reinforced by her belief, acquired early, internalized and then made largely inaccessible to consciousness, that men are powerful and that women cannot intervene. We should remember at this point just how much in society reinforces and reaffirms such a view, as the next chapter will show. The power bases in Western society are universally male-dominated, and women have had, and are still having, enormous struggles to make inroads and interventions into this male world. In the context of all this, it is perhaps hardly surprising that Suzanne was so depressed.

Third, there were factors relating to her mother, who had only recently grown older than Suzanne's grandmother had been at the time of her death. Ever since her grandmother's death Suzanne had had what she called 'strange feelings' which she was gradually able to identify. She was concerned in case her mother died without having talked with Suzanne about her grandmother's death. There was too much unfinished business. Much more traumatically, her mother's ageing unleashed a powerful and frightening grief reaction, which had been neither expressed nor recognized for thirty years. Additionally – and this relates to her return to full-time study – Suzanne came to realize that while her mother had always, on one level at least, encouraged her to pursue a career, this had not been an unequivocal message. She began to see that her own success was threatening to her mother. There was the unspoken implication that her own success would somehow be viewed as a betrayal and rejection of her mother's way of life.

The developing therapeutic relationship

These were the major strands of Suzanne's life history which she and her therapist were able to reassemble during the eighteen months in which they met. It was not an easy process. It was sometimes stormy, and often painful for Suzanne; and at times it was anxiety-provoking for her therapist as she tried to weather the storms, and to ensure Suzanne's safety while she was battling within them.

Therapy moved through different stages. As I have already indicated, in the early weeks Suzanne's primary feeling towards her therapist was one of relief and gratitude that someone was listening to her and taking her seriously. Her therapist felt a good working relationship had been created, one which Suzanne felt safe within, and within which she could start to explore the difficult areas that were gradually being identified. These first few weeks also saw considerable discussion between the two of them about how Suzanne might cope with her depression. One important part of taking her seriously was acknowledging the severity of her feelings and helping her to develop a system to cope with them.

As Suzanne came to regard therapy as a safe place, so she began to see that her present experiences were in fact linked to past events, and to past feelings, although, of course, they were also to do with present-day realities. As she looked at her past in more detail, and began to make more sense of it, so she started to experience and relive in therapy some of those earlier situations. But this time around she was able to attach to them the feelings and fears that had lain dormant and unrecognized for so many years. The expression of such feelings, so long locked away, their acceptance within the therapeutic relationship, and the identification of where they really belonged, enabled Suzanne to incorporate into herself those parts that had previously been denied entry.

For a long while, issues of trust and dependency were central in working with Suzanne. As we have seen, Suzanne was unsure about trusting anyone – she had been let down badly on too many occasions. She wanted to trust her therapist, but at the same time was frightened of doing so. Similarly, she had ambivalent feelings about dependency. Part of her felt very needy and just wanted to 'lean'; another part of her was terrified of this; while still another part of her was furious with her therapist for 'stirring up' these feelings within her. On many occasions she became very angry: her therapist was no good; it was just a job to her; she did not really care; she was giving her so little that it made no difference, and so on. Sometimes Suzanne would move rapidly from extreme rage to extreme distress; she would find it difficult to leave the room at the end of sessions; and she could be very anxious between sessions that her therapist would 'desert' her. It became very important that the therapist not only calmly tolerated and accepted such powerful feelings, but also that she was able to stand back and help Suzanne make sense of them, and understand their origins.

Anxieties about separations and endings were also central to the process. When they were at their height, Suzanne would often miss appointments, come late, or request a change of time at short notice. It was as though she was pre-empting the possibility of her therapist not being there while at the same time testing her to see whether she could really be trusted. She might even have been trying to create a self-fulfilling prophecy that 'if I push her hard enough she won't see me again and that will prove that she can't be trusted either'. Once Suzanne was able to make some sense of this, and to see her response to her therapist as intimately related to past relationships, it was possible for her to move forward from this position.

Unexpressed grief over her childhood losses formed another significant stage of the relationship between client and therapist. At times it was like having an anguished, confused and angry five-year-old in the room, although undoubtedly her most powerful expression of repressed grief came when, for the first time ever, she was able to look at the death of her grandmother when she was thirteen. For some weeks she often seemed more like an adolescent, and the grief-stricken Suzanne of that age was actively present in the sessions. It was difficult sometimes for the therapist to help Suzanne recover her adult self sufficiently before she left the room. But the adult Suzanne, in the midst of all her grief, still had to cope with her present world, and this involved the reality of caring for an actual adolescent daughter as well as a younger child. The expression of her grief within the context of a therapeutic relationship, that was not going to be destroyed or overwhelmed by angry or desperate feelings, was at times intensely painful for Suzanne. Finally, however, she was able to experience a new feeling of peace and ease within herself. A tempestuous storm had been ridden. Neither she nor her therapist had been irreparably damaged by it.

Throughout this process of work with Suzanne it was evident

to her therapist that careful ending of therapy was going to be of crucial importance. Given Suzanne's history of depression, the ending had to be linked to other losses and separations, and it was vital that this particular ending should not feel like another desertion to her. It had to be a loss about which she could express her feelings, and with which she could deal in a new way. The ending of therapy became the focus of thought and discussion a long while before it became a reality. In this way Suzanne and her therapist were able to look together at the meaning for her of the ending of therapy, to look at previous endings, to see how the present one could be different, to acknowledge the sad feelings, but also value the sense of moving on and that progress had been made. Good experiences stay inside us; they do not go away. They can be used, and referred back to when needed.

Suzanne's therapy shows how one client and her therapist were able to look at the contents of the 'locked box' that lay within her. Hers was in many ways an undramatic life story, not charged as some of my later examples are, with the power of abuse, anorexia or violence. Nevertheless her history has a power of its own and demonstrates the unhappiness that can exist hidden within conventional family life. There were, in addition, other layers, some of them related to the histories of her grandmother and mother, which as yet I have only touched upon. It is these which I look at in the next chapter, since they tell us more about the way patterns repeat themselves through different generations. Their stories also demonstrate how in some respects the position of women has changed (although in other respects it has not) over the last hundred years; and help us to understand how women who seek help from therapists and counsellors come to be where they are.

2

Three generations: the life of a family

Time past and time future
What might have been and what has been
Point to one end, which is always present.

T.S. Eliot

To understand the position and experiences of women today it is necessary to know something of their history. As we have seen, for Suzanne to make sense of herself, she needed to look at her own past. In the same way, the past, in a wider historical sense, must be recognized if we are to understand the conflicts and difficulties that women undergo. Women do not exist in a vacuum they are influenced by a society that both implicitly and explicitly gives messages about their expected and accepted role and position. As we shall come to see, these messages frequently have little to do with the well-being of women, but much more to do with what suits society in political and economic terms at a particular point in its development. Thus women are at the whim of changes that they are not able to control. These take place in the context of a society in which the political and economic structures are controlled and dominated by men. Even in this day and age the inroads made by women into these male bastions are limited, and yet it is there that decisions are made which exert enormous influence over the everyday lives of women.

To try to review the whole history of women is quite obviously a huge task, and one that could take us back many centuries. While trying to unravel the story of Suzanne, reference was made to her mother and grandmother, both very significant people in her life. Her grandmother was born in 1890. Although any starting date for examining women's history is inevitably somewhat arbitrary, the time of her birth is a good starting point. It will illustrate how the life of one family, of three generations of women, has been influenced by the events and developments of their time. Particular attention needs to be given to the role of women as workers, both in the home and in paid employment; to developments in education; and to changes in legislation relating to women's rights. As will be seen the effect of two world wars in this period had far reaching consequences extending way beyond the actual years of conflict.

This attempt to examine historically the world of women, leads us to ask where women are in the world of today. Have things really changed for them, or are all the old conflicts still really there albeit in slightly different form? Do women occupy a more central role in the power base of society? Where are they employed, and what are they doing? What is their economic position? To help explore this, we will return to the story of Suzanne, to look at her life, and at what is different for her, compared to the two generations before her. We will also examine the patterns that run through the lives of all three generations; aspects that have not changed; ways of relating; and experiences that may have affected them all in similar ways across the twentieth century.

The first generation: the story of Alice

Suzanne's grandmother, Alice, was born in 1890. The industrial revolution was in full swing; the male workforce was increasingly organizing itself into trade unions; the extent of poverty, both urban and rural, came under scrutiny from social reformers. Compulsory elementary education for boys and girls up to the age of twelve was now enforceable by law. Education for girls firmly prepared them for their future role as wives and mothers, and for most women employment outside the home was short term. Long-term prospects were irrelevant and generally inconceivable. Two Acts of Parliament gave married women the same rights to property as unmarried women. London University was admitting women students, although few women were able to use this opportunity. There were changes occurring at this time that are historically and politically significant. However, for the majority of women, their role in the world remained clearly and un-questionably defined: they were firmly rooted in the home and responsible for all childcare and domestic duties. This was in the context of the man being seen as the sole breadwinner, thereby carrying the weight of economic power. Working-class married women struggled within a web of appalling levels of poverty; housing of the most basic kind; infant mortality rates that made the death of a child commonplace; and an ethos that gave the 'worker' in the household the lion's share of the available food. Moreover, the assumption that working-class men could earn a 'family wage', that is, enough to support the whole family, was for many a myth. Women, therefore, often had to turn to casual and badly paid work to supplement a poor wage, thus struggling with the burden of two jobs, still familiar to women today.

For the middle-class woman the picture was different: if she worked prior to marriage her employment tended to be more pleasant and more protected. After marriage, although restricted within the confines of the home, she nevertheless enjoyed a higher standard of living. Labour was cheap and easily available, and the role of the middle-class woman was to supervise the smooth running of the home. Her participation in this process was limited; she did not dirty her own hands, ensuring that others did so on her behalf. The higher up the social scale, the more indirect a woman's involvement in this process. The upper classes employed a vast number of domestic servants (in itself one of the major sources of employment of young working-class women) and there was a complex hierarchy of status among the servants of these establishments. The picture of the languishing lady on the *chaise-longue*, so beloved of Victorian literature, perhaps reflects the fact that for many women in this situation a pale, interesting and seemingly passive persona was one identity that was easily open to them.

Suzanne's grandmother was born into a middle-class family, and as a child she never knew poverty. It was a comfortable life, although not outstandingly prosperous. She was one of five children, but even in this relatively affluent household one was to die in his first year of life. Suzanne remembered Alice telling her about the two young maids who were employed, and recounted her astonishment when as a young child she heard of the drudgery of their lengthy daily routine. Like other girls and boys of that time, Alice attended school until the age of twelve. She remembered long hours when the girls had to do needlework, the emphasis in those days being firmly on domestic subjects. She left school in 1902, at a time when the women's suffrage movement was gaining momentum, although at the age of twelve she was largely unaware of its existence and certainly unaware of its significance.

Alice's life fell into a predictable pattern in her early post-school years. She did not work, and her family did not intend her to do so. However, the ill health of her father forced a change in her circumstances, and she became employed as a milliner's assistant. Her employment was short-lived; as she later recalled the events of the time, her relief at giving up work was very evident when she married at eighteen. In her terms, at least for the time being, the status quo had been re-established. She did not feel she should be employed outside the home; she experienced this as a real insult to her rightful place in the world. For Alice, both social acceptance and self-acceptance lay in being in charge of her own household with a husband who would support her financially. Those were the days when middle-class married women normally did not work unless circumstances absolutely forced them to, and although there were some important regional variations, working-class women preferred not to. As we have seen, this preference did not reflect the reality for many. Work outside the home was generally a response to poverty, and not to choice.

Alice's only child, Suzanne's mother, Emily, was born in 1916. In 1917 disaster struck this young family, as it did so many others. Alice's husband was killed in action in the First World War, just one of the vast number of young men who were slaughtered in that conflict. Suzanne remembered vividly her grandmother's accounts of the despair she felt at the time: her growing disillusion with the war; her experience of real poverty for the first time in her life; her fear that she would always be alone as she could not envisage remarrying. With such huge losses of life such fears were real for many women. Following the war one in three women had to become self-supporting.

The effects of the First World War (and, similarly, as we shall come to see, of the Second) on the status and position of women were far-reaching. With the mass exodus of men leaving for war service, the country lost its supply of labour at a time when it was essential that industrial output was effectively maintained. Consequently, the view, so righteously upheld in pre-war days, that a woman's place was in the home, at first wavered, then crumbled, and soon gave way to the equally fervent expression of belief in women as workers.

While men were tempted and cajoled by patriotic outpourings to become cannon fodder, so women were tempted and cajoled into the workplace; what was previously banned now beckoned. Women became the workforce that maintained the heaviest of heavy industry: they built armaments; they maintained and tarred roads; they did many of the jobs that had previously belonged in the male domain. And, they were, of course, still mothers. During the war women carried out 90 per cent of the work normally done by men; they discovered abilities and uncovered potential previously unrecognized. However, this process was not one of gradual self-discovery. It was imposed by political and economic factors. Suddenly, and conveniently, women were discovered to be made of sterner stuff. But only temporarily. At the end of the war all the women workers were dismissed.

For Alice, life as a widow was hard. She struggled to bring up her daughter in an economic climate in which many prices had doubled in the war years. Women who, like her, were trying to survive on a small and fixed income, fought a continual battle against poverty and, ultimately, against destitution. At the end of the war the dreaded Poor Law was still in force, representing for many the end of the road in the battle to stay respectable. Alice, however, was never entirely destitute: she had a small income, and her skills in millinery offered her some earning potential. Her memories were those of poverty, but she was well off compared to many around her. Her child never went without clothes or shoes; and they only occasionally had insufficient food. She saw many around her who suffered more. In the years following the war most women returned to the home. Their foray into active participation in the wider world had been but brief. Many found themselves in the same position as Alice; their husbands were dead, and the status of war hero was both short-lived and did not feed hungry mouths. Moreover, although so many women, both single and widowed, now faced a life alone, with little hope of marriage, the prevailing and powerful view taken by society was that a woman needed a man to take care of her.

Some changes were occurring. The 1918 Representation of the People Act gave the vote to certain categories of women over the age of thirty. It gave the vote to all men over the age of twenty-one. Many women who had taken over, without prior training or warning, the running of essential services during the war years were now deemed to lack the maturity necessary for full suffrage. The battle for suffrage continued, and was finally won in 1928.

In 1922 the first woman Member of Parliament was elected, and in the same year the Law of Property Act was passed, for the first time giving wives and daughters equal rights in intestacy cases with fathers and sons. The following year saw another major piece of legislation: the Matrimonial Act made the grounds for divorce the same for women as they were for men.

In the field of education, some movement was also evident. In the private sector a small number of fee-paying schools were established, offering a wide-ranging curriculum, with an accompanying ethos of educational opportunity that was not reflected in state provision. In state schools the emphasis remained very firmly on subjects that would equip girls suitably for a domestic role; indeed the 1926 Board of Education report recommended that there should be more housecraft on the syllabus for girls. In 1920 women were able to take degrees at Oxford (Cambridge resisted this move until 1948) although only a very small number actually did so.

The second generation: the story of Emily

Alice was thirty-eight years of age, and her daughter, Emily, twelve when women were finally given full voting rights. Alice, although not a political militant of her time, remembered this as a great victory. Emily was brought up in the firm knowledge that many women had fought long and hard for this basic right. Her childhood and youth was in many ways different from her mother's. She was an only child in a single-parent family that struggled to keep poverty at bay. Her education was more extensive than her mother's, and undertaken in the knowledge that she would have to support herself financially until the marriage that she hoped for. She stayed at school until she was fourteen and did very well, but there was no possibility of continuing in full-time education. However, she did undertake some further part-time evening study. In the midst of a political climate marked by economic depression, rising unemployment, and consequent pressure for women either to stay at home or to enter the traditional realms of domestic service, Emily managed to find clerical work.

In comparison with the wages a man earned, Emily was very badly paid. Although the trade unions had grown in membership and strength in the inter-war years, they were generally not only uninterested in the rights of women, but had a powerful vested interest in keeping women out of employment. During these years when the trade union movement membership was almost entirely male, both the economic depression and the availability of cheap female labour cast an unwelcome shadow over their hard-won victories. They were not sympathetic to the plight of women: they were too great a threat to an already vulnerable position.

Emily enjoyed her job, and remained in employment until her marriage in 1937. In common with most women of that time, she then automatically gave up her job. There were some class and regional differences, but generally marriage still meant returning to the role of housewife; indeed, some occupations still imposed a marriage bar. Again, it was a war that not only dramatically disrupted family life but also forced the roles of women to undergo a major shift. Just as in the First World War, sudden changes in thinking resulted from political and economic pressures and were powerfully imposed. War temporarily opened doors for many women, but not in response to their needs. It was a response to the requirements and demands of a wartime economy.

From 1937 until 1943 Emily stayed at home. She cared for her husband and for her daughter, Suzanne, born in 1941. She was responsible for running the home. Soon after the start of the war her husband left for active service and was only home on leave for brief periods. As in many other families, Emily's mother moved into the family home to be with her daughter. When Emily responded to the call that 'there is a job awaiting every woman' and returned to work, Alice happily took over the care of her little granddaughter. Of course, many women returning to work at this time did not have relatives available for childcare. This was not the obstacle it would have been in pre-war years. Once again a major ideological transformation occurred: the advent of war was accompanied, conveniently, by the simultaneous discovery that alternative care was not harmful to small children! Crèches and nurseries were organized, and a variety of social provision encouraged women to work. As in the First World War, women demonstrated that they could and would do any job, and that, at the same time, they could care for home and children.

Emily enjoyed her job. In later years she was to tell her daughter: 'I felt whole again, and not guilty, because during the war we were supposed to work.' But she did not enjoy the same wages as a man would have done, for women's pay was still low. In the war years there was some negotiation on wages with the unions, resulting in agreements that after six months a woman doing the same job as a man should be paid the same. However, such agreements, although establishing a principle, did not work well in practice. It was too easy for employers to adopt avoiding tactics, and many did. Women working in the Women's Land Army may have felt very well off in comparison with those who worked on farms before the war. They earned double the peacetime rate, but it was still half that of men.

With the conclusion of the war in 1945, this further taste of the wider world ended for many women. During the war the message was that their country needed them; now it was that their home and family should be their firm priority. Crèches and nurseries were closed, often with very little warning. Mothers and their children were faced with a change in policy that was arbitrary and non-negotiable. Doors were shut on them with little or no regard to their real needs. Women had once more served their purpose; they could now retreat to their homes quietly and without fuss.

Once again the message was clear: young children needed their mothers. The work of John Bowlby[1] left many with the firm understanding that even brief separations could damage their children. Bowlby's work, and the conclusions he reached, were based on studies of children in institutional care, but became generalized to all children. At a time when there was such societal pressure to return to the home, the work of Bowlby was conveniently timed. The dual pressure from a government that dictated the rights of returning heroes to employment, and from a childcare expert who argued that anything other than full-time maternal devotion could lead to delinquency, were indeed powerful. To resist these two simultaneous injunctions without falling into a whirlpool of guilt and anxiety was too much for most women, and the back-to-the-home policy proved effective.

Emily, like many others, gave up her job and returned to working in the home. Her husband took up his previous employment, and Emily's mother left to live separately, albeit nearby. In 1946 Suzanne started school and a year later her baby sister was born. To an outsider it may well have appeared that a coherent and stable family structure had been easily and comfortably re-established after considerable, but temporary, upheaval during the war period.

But, as Suzanne's own story has shown, this external appearance was not matched by the internal perceptions of at least some of the family members. These transitions were particularly problematic for Suzanne, and were remembered as such. She also remembered this time as one of unhappiness for both her grandmother and her mother. In all likelihood it was not an easy time for her father either. It must have appeared to him, and this is perhaps supported in reality, that he had disrupted a female trio that had managed quite well without him.

This picture is the other side of the one more commonly presented of the returning hero being rapturously received back into the welcoming bosom of the family. Such enormous disruptions to family life as was caused by both world wars could not be easily put aside. The traditional roles of women had been challenged; it had been acknowledged that changes could occur, and that they could be incorporated into the other demands of home and childcare. The knowledge of the possibility of a different way of being could not be entirely wiped out, although the post-war period certainly submerged this to a quite considerable, and entirely intentional, extent.

With the end of the war came major political changes that were almost revolutionary in their impact. A wealth of legislation marked the onset of the welfare state which was impressive in both its aims and extent. This is not the place to examine in detail the breadth of these changes, although to understand the world that Suzanne and other women of her time were brought up in it is necessary to identify the central strands of policy changes. One of the most significant changes was the introduction of free health-care. Women came forward for treatment with complaints that they had previously had to tolerate if they could not afford to pay. In many families it was the breadwinner's health that had to be protected, and surviving on a low income left little to pay for treatment of 'women's complaints'. Women were used to being bottom of the pile when it came to sharing scarce resources, whether it be food or doctor's fees. Consequently, the intro-duction of the National Health Service in 1948 benefited them, and their children, enormously.

The introduction of Family Allowances in 1946 was another measure that directly benefited women. These were paid for each child after the first and were funded from national taxation, that is, they were not based on insurance contributions. After a free vote in the House of Commons it was decided that the Family Allowance should be payable to the mother, and not to the father. This acknowledgement that women had a right to control of this money was an important step; for some it was their only access to finance other than that given them by their husbands.

Changes in the education system were also much in evidence at this time. The 1944 Education Act, and the formation of a government ministry with responsibility for education, repre-sented a major policy shift. For the first time a universal system of education for all children up to the age of fifteen was introduced. Further education was also included in this plan, with the provision of financial assistance where necessary. Traditionally, girls' education had been viewed as less important than the education of boys, who were destined from an early age to be breadwinners and decision-makers. What, after all, was the purpose of educating girls when all they were going to do was to become housewives and mothers? This created a somewhat circular argument, and one that was difficult to escape from. However, the 1944 Education Act at least ensured that all girls received education to a specified age, and did greatly increase their chances of continuing thereafter. What it did not do was to remove the subject and attitude discrepancy, which, as will be seen later, still exists.

The third generation: the story of Suzanne

Born as she was in 1941, the world Suzanne entered as a child and teenager was in many ways very different from that experienced by her mother and grandmother before her. How great these changes really were, or whether the underlying situation for women now is really the old one in disguise, we shall attempt to clarify. There were some obvious and important changes. Whereas her mother's education stopped at fourteen, and her grandmother's at twelve, Suzanne continued in full-time education until she was twenty-one and throughout that time she received financial support from the state.

The boom in the 'new' universities in the 1960s benefited her, as it did so many other middle-class girls. It is worth pointing out that in 1963, when Suzanne was completing her studies, the Newson Report[2] was suggesting that for the academically less able girls the emphasis should be on home-making skills. Not so, of course, for the academically less able boys. The distinctions in girls' subjects and boys' subjects remained very clear. In the same year, 25 per cent of all university entrants were girls, although very few were entering the 'traditional' male disciplines of science and technology.

Of the three generations of women in this one family, Suzanne had the longest and most easily accessible education. This in turn enabled her to move more smoothly into a career, although she still opted for one that has traditionally been viewed as acceptable for women. Indeed, Suzanne remembers teaching being given the seal of approval when she was a pupil at school. Teaching was very much encouraged as a career that ultimately would fit in with a girl's other role in life, that of being a wife and a mother. She was brought up with the assumption that one day she would marry, and that if she were to continue to pursue a career it would essentially need to fit in with these other commitments.

Yet, simultaneously, there was another pressure, that she was fortunate and privileged to have access to an education that had been denied her mother and her grandmother. Consequently, she must be grateful and not waste the opportunities presented to her; she must be successful, and always work hard. Perhaps the hidden injunction that lay beneath the obvious messages was one that is recognizable to many women of Suzanne's generation. It is rarely made explicit but often felt to be there: be successful, but not too successful; be ambitious, but cautiously so; be careful not to be too competitive with men; their male powers will be easily threatened.

Additionally, there was some fear about succeeding where her mother had not. On the one hand, a girl's academic success can evoke maternal pride; but, on the other, it can also be experienced as disloyalty to, and rejection of, a mother's accepted values, so leading to feelings of isolation in the daughter. Increased opportunity for Suzanne, while it freed her from some of the constraints experienced by earlier generations, did not make her life conflict-free or straightforward.

Other developments, too, had their significance for Suzanne's generation. The wider availability of contraception and the legalizing of abortion gave women greater control over their lives and bodies in a way that was unimaginable to earlier generations. While women still largely take responsibility for domestic tasks, the technological advances and the advent of convenience foods has at least lightened the load. Family size is smaller; infant mortality rates have declined; childhood illnesses have been rendered less severe with the availability of more sophisticated medical treatment.

Legislative changes

The 1970s and 1980s have seen the introduction of a considerable amount of legislation broadly aimed at reducing the inequalities between men and women in some key areas. The effectiveness of such legislative changes is always in question. Changing the law does not automatically change attitudes, yet without changes in attitude legislation is hard to enforce. Perhaps a degree of good will and positive intention is assumed to exist within society when such legal changes are made. More cynically, and perhaps more accurately, creating legislation may be the end in itself: it can be a response to pressure from powerful or vociferous groups; it can be pointed to as a genuine attempt to deal with a problem, while in reality it contains so many loopholes as to render it ineffective.

Individual attempts to enforce and utilize legislation are fraught with difficulty. The 1970 Equal Pay Act is a prime example of legislation that was impressive in name, though ineffective in practice. This Act only applied to work that was equivalent for men and women and was therefore very limited in scope. Very few women came within its ambit, and where they did it was an easy task for employers to alter the work slightly so that it was no longer equivalent. The Act blatantly failed to achieve what its title suggested it would do. It was not until 1984, prompted by the European Court of Justice, that the Act was amended so that women could get equal pay for work of equal value. Even with that important amendment it remained unclear whether the large number of women employed in exclusively female jobs, often with low pay, would benefit.

Other legislation has also been significant. Changing employment laws gave women the right to paid maternity leave. It also gave them the right to return to work after the birth of their child, opening up the possibility of continuous employment that was previously denied. This is a far cry from the days, not so long ago, when most women automatically gave up their jobs on marriage. Indeed, in 1987 women made up 42 per cent of the workforce in Britain, although their growing equality numerically was not reflected in their earnings or their type of employment. In terms of their average gross weekly earnings, women took home approximately two-thirds of a man's wage, a gap that has persisted in spite of the amendment to the Equal Pay Act. This differential is only partly explained by the fact of poor pay in occupations mainly staffed by women. For example, while two-thirds of laboratory technicians are men, women in the same job still only earn 80 per cent of a man's wage; again, while half of those employed as footwear workers are men, the women still earn just under 70 per cent of what is earnt by men.

Women as paid workers: where are they?

The positions women hold in work are also significant. In the political arena the UK in the 1980s still only had one woman cabinet member (the Prime Minister). Only 6 per cent of Members of Parliament are women.[3] Schoolteaching, traditionally an area women have been encouraged to enter, demonstrates enormous inequalities. In nursery and primary education about 80 per cent of teachers are women, and in the secondary sector it is about 50 per cent: yet they are concentrated in the lower grades. Men are four times as likely to become headteachers. In the universities this situation is even more pronounced: in 1986–7 only 3 per cent of professors and only 8 per cent of senior lecturers were women.

Similarly, in the English judiciary, in 1987 out of seventy-six High Court judges only three were women. Although many more women are entering both the legal and the medical professions, they continue to be underrepresented at the most senior levels. In 1985, 39 per cent of general practitioners aged under thirty, and 25 per cent of all hospital doctors, were women, and in the same year 15 per cent of practising solicitors were women. However, only 13 per cent of women reached consultant grade in hospitals, and only 7 per cent became partners in solicitors' practices.

In British industry the picture is even more pronounced: less than 0.5 per cent of company chairpersons are women, and they constitute just over 6 per cent of senior managers. Within the Civil Service, traditionally a major employer of women, they constitute 70 per cent of clerical assistants; 5 per cent of under-secretaries, and there are no women permanent secretaries. Taking a more global view: women are half the population; they do nearly two-thirds of the world's work, and yet they earn just one-tenth of the world's income.

Currently, yet another shift is taking place in government attitudes towards women in employment. In January 1989 a junior employment minister stated that women would be desperately needed in the workforce as the number of available young people declined. (No prizes for guessing what the current policy might be if the number of young people in the workforce were not declining!) At the same time government assistance in funding childcare is severely limited allowing tax relief on work place nursery provision. And with so many more women working it may seem reasonable to assume that the burden of household tasks would be more fairly distributed. Not so: a recent survey carried out by the Family Policy Studies Centre points out that 'while it is true that men – on average – probably take a more active role in the home than in the past, this is typically a helping role rather than an egalitarian allocation of domestic responsibility'.[4] It is still the woman who is responsible for looking after the home; the man may assist, but he does no more. Even when both partners work full-time, the majority of the women are left with the bulk of household tasks as their clear responsibility.

Over three generations, women's role in the labour market, and their role within the home and as mothers, has seen considerable movement, but also vacillation, in terms of government policies and objectives. Women have been used as a back-up labour force when economically and politically necessary, while at other times they have been firmly relegated to the home. Not only has this been confusing to women, adding another layer to the contradictory role demands which many of them experience, but also it has had the effect of casting doubts on the value of motherhood and mothering. Society's ambivalence regarding women's employment, and the lack of real support for mothers, have combined powerfully together with the false, packaged image of ideal motherhood, frequently seen in the media and advertising. The result has been a mixture of messages impossible to disentangle or to make sense of. Policies towards women could fairly be described as a somewhat arbitrary mess of political expedience, false idealization, and cavalier attitudes all taking place within the context of a society in which the power base lies firmly with men.

It is this world that Suzanne and others of her generation find themselves in, a world that is in some ways vastly different from that of her mother's and grandmother's generations. Women's role is no longer so firmly fixed in the home; they can control their own fertility to a greater extent; abortion is a real choice; divorce and single parenthood do not carry the same stigma as they once did; education is more easily available, and even though housework is still firmly left with the vast majority of women it is not the same drudgery that it was for earlier generations. Women are organizing themselves and taking charge of their lives in new ways; many are more assertive and more militant. Groups such as Women's Aid and Women for Peace, rape crisis centres, women's therapy centres, the active involvement of women in the miners' strike, the Greenham women – all suggest women's growing confidence that they have a voice and that they can be heard. Many may feel that this voice is not being adequately heard, and that there is a long way to go. Certainly, in other ways change is not so apparent. The figures on employment quoted above should not be underestimated in their significance. They clearly indicate that in the power structures of the UK men are disproportionately overrepresented. Some argue that women's real influence lies in their role as home-maker and carer. While the value of that is clear, it is not reflected in society's treatment of women who occupy that role. That has not changed.

Towards a broader understanding

To understand individual women in therapy and counselling, a counsellor also has to understand both their wider history, and their current position in society. Some may ask why we need this view when therapy and counselling deals with individuals. It is because a counsellor's concern is to stay close to the experience of an individual in her own world – a world that is part of the larger world, which is influenced by political, economic and social issues. The experience and perceptions of an individual come not only from inside her, but also from outside her. Internal worlds meet external worlds; external worlds exert powerful pressures and demands that cannot be dismissed or ignored, without rendering part of the picture invisible. When women try to express their conflicts, and their unhappiness, and try to untangle the complexity of strands of their lives, it is demeaning or arrogant if their therapist is not able to acknowledge the real pressures and real contradictions they are also facing.

Equally, however, there is always the temptation, just as unhelpful, to brush away the psychological aspects of individual sorrow and suffering by saying that 'it's all society's fault'. To do so equally demeans the weight and significance of an individual's own life, history and dynamics. In the same way as emphasis on the purely societal or political level can block exploration of the psychological, the reverse is also true. With any client we are dealing with a very complex series of interactions, often with no clear cut lines between them. That needs to be acknowledged before there can be any attempt at unravelling. As Suzanne has shown, her present distress and her own past history are closely linked.

Having seen how changes in society have influenced three generations, another question remains. What similarities are there in the lives of the three women: Alice, Emily and Suzanne? Are there any patterns that are repeated throughout the generations? It is striking that all three women had to cope with the absence of their husband. For Alice this temporary absence during war turned to a permanent one on his death. She had to support herself and her child at a time when this was particularly difficult, with little support, and with little acknowledgement of the hardship. She had to cope with grief, with isolation, with poverty, and with the double demands of caring for a young child while supporting her financially. This was true of many women at this time. Yet very little heed has been given to this suffering, compared to the attention paid to the vast loss of men on the battlefields.

Similarly, Emily lost her husband to war, although for her the separation was not permanent. The war involved other separations: leaving her young daughter to return to work does not appear to have been traumatic for either of them, but leaving her employment, and the departure of her mother when her husband returned were difficult times for her. They were also, as we have seen, difficult for Suzanne. Again it seems that these problems were not given any credence by anyone. Men were welcomed home and were given back their jobs. Some protection and acknowledgement was thereby afforded to men, but little to women. Having made the shift to employment and independence with little choice, they were thrust back into domesticity with even less choice. Men were applauded for their war victory; an accolade awaited them. Did anyone applaud the women?

Suzanne did not lose her husband to war, but she did lose him, on many occasions, to his job. She lost him to a world of work that was male-dominated, and to which she did not have equal access. Her earlier equality was lost, but, as with her mother and grandmother, the difficulties imposed by the situation were not acknowledged. Although there are obvious differences between the three generations, these women shared a common experience: of seeing men come and go, and doing 'important' things that women were apparently unable to do; of not complaining, since it is important that men fight wars and make money: of having to be flexible and adaptable. They were expected to praise their menfolk – as having paid the ultimate price, as returning heroes, or as providers for their women and children.

Another common feature, manifested in different ways in the different generations, was experienced by all three women: women are often caught up in processes and events created by decisions made by men. Women, correctly see themselves as playing a central role; at the same time, they recognize that they are unable to assert much control over policies, or over the outcome of policies. Although they lack control, they are deeply affected by many of the consequences. They carry responsibilties and burdens in a manner that is largely unseen and given little credit. On the contrary, the role of men carries greater visibility and is much more obviously given credit. The availabillty of employment and education were crucial to Alice, Emily, and

Suzanne, although they had little control over these areas. Suzanne may have had access to education and to employment inconceivable in earlier generations, but it is also clear that at school she was encouraged to enter a profession that would also accommodate the roles of wife and mother. Although the world of employment was open to her, as a mother she still had somehow to merge two worlds. In the same way, her grandmother had needed somehow to combine the two. During the war years Suzanne's mother had done the same, although her job was then to be taken away from her.

Although there were differences for the three of them, there is an underlying pattern that is uncomfortably similar. First, for these women, as for many others, domestic and working worlds were not rigidly defined or divided. They overlapped, and sometimes conflicted, but essentially somehow had to fit together, even if in tension. A major consideration for all three in their working lives was how work would fit in with their children. Suzanne's grandmother, after her husband's death, had to work. Her work had to fit in around childcare. When Emily worked, Alice was there to be the carer. Suzanne chose a job with hours and holidays to suit her school-age children, although this did not remove all the conflicts. And her husband did not have to make such compromises: he was free to take a job that meant absences from home. Absences to fight a war are obviously not quite the same, nevertheless they reinforce the pattern of it being acceptable for a man to go away; for a woman to stay at home and take sole responsibility, and for her in effect to do two jobs simultaneously. For the three generations employment was not a matter of clear choice and preference: it depended on circumstances into which Alice, Emily, and Suzanne in turn had to fit.

Another pattern that is evident for all generations is that of separation and loss. Obviously in every life there are deaths, losses, and separations; but in this particular family there were many, combined with an ongoing difficulty both in acknowledging them and in dealing with the resulting grief. The effects on Suzanne of these losses were deep; although, equally, her grandmother suffered similarly at the death of her husband. She, too, had felt very alone during that period of her life, her grief had been enormous yet unrecognized, and she had faced huge practical difficulties. Emily, her daughter, as a very young child lost a father whom she hardly knew. She was too young to grieve for him, but not too young to experience the effects of her mother's grief.

Perhaps this very early experience – although, of course, not consciously remembered – partly accounted for the enormous grief she felt in later years when her own mother, Suzanne's grandmother, died. At this time, too, Suzanne experienced the most enormous loss, unrecognized by those around her. As a young girl she experienced the same isolation in her grief, as her grandmother as a young woman, and her mother as a young child, had felt all those years earlier.

To understand something of the experience of today's woman, we need to know something about the experience of yesterday's. We need to have some awareness of how society has developed and how the role of women within that society has been defined, and by whom. This must never detract from the necessity of listening with care to the story of each individual woman, and must not minimize her significance and value as a unique person in her own right. It does, however, place her story in context, thus increasing the breadth of our understanding, and making available further insights. To comprehend the many layers of the person, we need, first, to know and accept that person as an individual; second, to look at the history of the family for further insights and third, to be aware of the wider society and its influences. Essentially, we need to encompass a multi-dimensional view so that we can avoid tunnel vision and its resulting distortions.

Notes

1 Bowlby, J. (1947). *Child Care and the Growth of Love*. Penguin.
2 Ministry of Education. Central Advisory Council for Education (England) (1963). *Half Our Future*. (Newson Report), HMSO.
3 The source of all the statistics on employment quoted in this chapter are: The Equal Opportunities Commission (1987). *Women and Men in Britain: a Statistical Profile*. HMSO; The Equal Opportunities Commission (1988). *Women and Men in Britain: a Research Profile*. HMSO.
4 Henwood, M., Rimmer, L. and Wicks, M. (1987). *Inside the Family: Changing Roles of Men and Women*. Family Policy Studies Centre.

3

Girls will be girls

What are little girls made of?
Sugar and spice
And all that's nice.
That's what little girls are made of.

What are little boys made of?
Snaps and snails
And puppy dog's tails.
That's what little boys are made of.

Traditional nursery rhyme

God created little girls
To cuddle in your arms
He made them warn and very soft
With sweet and gentle charms.

Now, sons aren't always angels
But when all is said and done
There's nothing more exciting
Than a brand new baby son.

Birth congratulations cards 1989

In our 'enlightened' culture terms such as 'sexism', 'equality of opportunity' and 'discrimination' are tossed casually around, part of our current vocabulary. As we have seen in the previous chapter, the degree to which any of this has been translated into action is in many ways disappointing. Girls and young women today are promised the open door, only to find, on closer inspection, that there are minefields that prevent them going any further. Older women, brought up with a clearer view of what their role should be, face other related difficulties. They, too, are challenged by the idea of the new woman, but they carry with them their own history. They have been firmly instructed in the old ways. Women of all ages grow up with a picture of what it means to be a woman. Some aspects of that picture have changed with the years; others have remained intact and unwavering. All girls and women are, to some extent, restrained by the boundaries that frame the picture.

How girls are brought up to see themselves, first as girls and later as women, is central to our undertanding of the issues women bring to therapy and counselling. As we have seen in Suzanne's case, she carried with her a history in which the personal and political were intricately intertwined. The messages she had received about herself came from many different directions and sources. Understanding these was essential to her discovery of herself.

Sexual differentiation is no accident. How girls should look, how they should behave, think, and feel, are closely linked to the economic and political structures of society at a given point in time. Sue Sharpe reminds us that:

> It is important to remember that sex differentiation and its surrounding attitudes and values does not develop in an arbitrary way. It is vitally influenced by the nature of the economic structure of a society and the division of labour that has been developed around it.[1]

It is clear that in wartime the stereotype of the strong, fit and fighting young man serves its purpose. Women can stay at home and mind the babies. Men can defend, do battle and kill. In time of shortfall in the labour force, in peace or in war, women can be workers, too. Yet the fit and fighting young man may be less popular when aggression is vented in the football crowd, and women wanting to work in times of high unemployment may cause an uncomfortable ripple politically. Although sexual stereotyping may have some problematic side-effects on a wider social scale, at the same time it successfully maintains the system. But on an individual level the disadvantages and losses are numerous. Childcare stays female-dominated, and the implications of this are considerable; positions of power and influence remain male-dominated. A wedge is pushed between the two sexes, and there arises a danger that masculine and feminine become opposite and opposing positions. With one side having the monopoly of power economically and politically, the potential for exploitation is obvious.

Messages about being a girl and being a woman come from many directions. Initially they come from parents, particularly the child's own mother, the active and present parent for most children in the early months and years. Correspondingly, messages will also be received from the father, via his role as the more absent parent who disappears regularly into a largely unseen, but obviously important, world. A small child soaks up a way of being from his/her surroundings in much the same way as blotting paper soaks up water. If it is a woman who cares for you, who responds to your needs, and to others, who is available and accessible, and who feeds and nurtures, then a powerful model of being a woman is presented for absorption. The model is further reinforced by the father who is not part of the immediate system, but evidently involved in another one, apparently unattainable to mother and you, but depicted as crucial to your well-being. What child has not heard the words: 'Daddy has to go out to work to earn money to look after us'? Children brought up in single-parent households (usually, of course, single mothers) have a different experience. Nevertheless, it is still the woman who occupies the caring role. There are still very few households in which roles are genuinely exchanged, or even really shared. We do not yet know how such households might affect a child's view of himself/ herself. Male unemployment may create the possibility of a greater paternal share in childrearing, but it would appear that the appalling pressures of being unemployed are unlikely to en- courage a positive attitude in most men to such an opportunity of more actively sharing in parenting.

From the earliest days then, a child's experience is of woman as mother and carer. Nancy Chodorow[2] states that 'women's mother- ing is one of the few universal and enduring elements of the sexual divisions of labour', and this is highly significant for the develop- ing awareness of both boys and girls. Even prior to birth a child's gender is of significance to the person who will be the primary carer, that is, the mother. Ann Oakley[3], in her study of mothers, found that before birth 22 per cent of mothers expressed a preference for a girl, and 54 per cent a boy. Following birth, 56 per cent of those with a girl were pleased; 44 per cent were disappointed. Of mothers with boys, 93 per cent were pleased, and only 7 per cent disappointed. She also found that 'daughters were likely to provoke less positive and more negative feelings in their mothers than sons'. It is easy to feel some indignation on behalf of these little girl babies who appear to be disadvantaged from the moment of birth, in terms of maternal attitude.

There is evidence that from very early days mothers treat girl and boy babies differently. H.A. Moss[4] found considerable differ- ences. Simply put, boys received more attention. They are held more than daughters, are given more overall attention, are stimulated to a greater extent, and looked at more. R. Hartley,[5] in a study of children aged one to five years, found similar differences in maternal treatment of boys and girls. Mothers, even of such young children, were concerned over the appearance of their daughters. They fussed over how they looked in a way that was not evident with boys. Children were focused towards gender-appropriate toys – girls to dolls; boys to cars and other more active toys. The content and style of language was related to the sex of the child. Older girls were expected to help with younger siblings and housework, while boys were not.

It is easy to dismiss the significance of maternal concern about appearance as a superficial issue. However, it suggests that from earliest experience of self-consciousness girls are told that it matters how they look. Inevitably, this affects how a girl acts, plays and behaves. Watching small children in a playground points to some obvious differences. Not only are boys encouraged to be more adventurous and to take more risks, but even their clothing facilitates this. With the advent of jeans and trainers for both sexes, some girls are now less restricted by what they wear. However, a large number remain dressed in clothing that make ease of movement difficult, and bring about grazed knees and maternal annoyance when the inevitable falls result in injuries to self, and to less than robust clothes. As girls grow older this is further emphasized. As they become more aware of their bodies, and of male reactions to them, skirts and dresses restrain even more their ability to run, jump and climb. Both attitudes and dress restrict girls from an early age to a less active and outgoing existence than their male counterparts.

Marianne Grabucker describes her attempts to bring up her small daughter without the gender conditioning that she feels is the result of centuries of patriarchy. Her account is outstanding in the way it details the daily life of a child and a mother. It illustrates clearly how, from many sources, girls are encouraged to be more passive, less active and less assertive than boys. It shows, both subtly and more obviously, how this situation is both generated and maintained by friends, family, nursery school teachers, and by popular images of women. She begins her book with the powerful assertion that her daughter

was not going to become like us, that is, women born in the post-war period. I did not want her to be compliant, to keep her opinions to herself, and to smile sweetly instead of contradicting. I did not want her to be always checking and rethinking her ideas before opening her mouth, unlike her male counterparts who would say everything three times and then repeat it once again.[6]

In the course of the three years in which her book was written the difficulty of achieving this desire, and effecting her belief, becomes very apparent. It is not easy to raise daughters differently in isolation. Attitudes towards boys need to move simultaneously. She concludes: 'only when both sexes from childhood on are engaged in a continual process of change, moving forward step by step, is there any hope for a future of real equality'.[7]

Other mothers of daughters will be familiar with many of the scenarios Grabucker describes. When my own older daughter was two, she was fearlessly and happily dangling from the top of a large climbing frame, enjoying herself immensely. In tones of admiration another mother said: 'She should have been born a boy, that one'. A third mother, apparently mistakenly interpreting my lack of intervention in terms of my advanced pregnancy, removed my indignant daughter 'in case she fell', leaving her own younger and rather less robust son to play uninterrupted. The influence of these kinds of comment and intervention should not be underestimated.

We see that, from their earliest days, conditioning of girls is well under way. To examine this process in more depth, it is valuable to explore various aspects of a girl's world, looking further at the significance of care by the mother; the role of the father; education; and the everyday environment which so subtly influences the attitudes and perceptions of a young child. What sense do girls and boys make of everything that is around them? What do they learn implicitly about how women and men are, in relation to one another and to the world around them? Through my experience of working with both children and adults, it becomes evident how impressions are conveyed, and statements explicitly made, which together direct girls and women into gender-specific ways of being. But though these may be specific ways of being, the messages that women receive make for confusion and restrictions.

Messages to girls and women: where they come from and what they say

Mothers and daughters

Boys and girls commonly identify with the parent of the same sex. The essential difference for girls is that for them this involves identifying with the parent who has been their primary carer. And just as girls identify with their mother, so mothers also identify with their daughters. They, too, have been daughters. They have a shared experience which they cannot have in their relationship with their sons. They know, too, that their daughter will learn from them how to be a mother herself. Certainly, for many women becoming a mother uncovers their own early experiences, sometimes in a startlingly vivid way. This essential difference is referred to by Nancy Chodorow as the 'double identification process': girls identifying with mothers, mothers with daughters. Of mothers, she says:

> Because they are the same gender as their daughters and have been girls, mothers of daughters tend not to experience these infant daughters as separate from them in the same way as do mothers of infant sons.[8]

Because of this, and reinforced firmly by the ever present stereotypes of active boys and passive girls, it becomes harder for women to allow their small daughters independence and a separate identity. At the same time a girl is caught in a dilemma. She must be like her mother to attain and retain her female identity; while in order to become separate and autonomous as an individual, she must also leave her mother. Small wonder that many women, when describing the agonies of this process, feel that their successful autonomy has been experienced as treachery by their mothers. Talking to women, it is evident that many are given an ambiguous message by their mother: 'be like me, but don't be like me'. Mothers may well experience a desire for life to be fuller and more independent for their daughters. At the same time they can feel this as a betrayal of their own way of life, which for them is synonomous with womanhood.

In some senses, the development of gender identity in young girls is a smoother process than it is for boys. There are certainly, as we shall come to see, plenty of role models around. Absent fathers, and a plethora of female carers, do not provide such easy access for boys. However, while it may be smoother, in that a continuous and available input is obviously in evidence, it is also more complex. A boy does not have to strive to be like his mother in order to assume a masculine identity, while simultaneously trying to separate from her. He is given every encouragement to join the male world, and is taught to believe that he has a right to be there.

The emphasis on motherhood equalling parenting has a lot to answer for. Dorothy Dinnerstein sees both sexes as the losers:

> Motherhood gives us boys that will grow reliably into childish men, unsure of their grasp on life's primitive realities. And it gives us girls who will grow reliably into childish women, unsure of their right to full worldly status. Such men and women can be relied upon to seek each other out, for they have proverbially complementary strengths and weaknesses.[9]

Some may feel that childish men would win in a final count, and they certainly have the edge in terms of actual power. However, it is well to remember that all can lose, and she goes on to suggest that:

> When men start participating as deeply as women in the initiation of infants into the human estate and when both male and female parents come to carry for all of us the special meanings of early childhood, the trouble we have reconciling these meanings with person-ness will finally be faced. The consequence, of course, will be a fuller and more realistic, a kinder and at the same time more demanding definition of person-ness.[10]

When women look back on their experiences of growing up, what do they remember about their relationship with their mother? Memories are, of course, various, but there are common themes that run across them. Talking to groups of women, it is evident that for them as small children mother was the one who was always there. She did everything in the house, and there was an emphasis on a meal being on the table when father returned at the end of a day. For most of these women, paid work outside the home came as children grew older. If they worked when they had young children, this somehow was fitted in around the children. A grandmother may have helped out with childcare, but the predominant memory was of a mother who was mainly home-based, and committed to home and child. In one group of women, several were aware that their own mother would have preferred a boy, backing up Ann Oakley's findings. One woman in her thirties said:

I know my mother wanted a boy. She used to tell me so. She used to say that as she'd had a girl, she wanted a pretty little thing, and somehow she got this big lump instead.

Another talked of her mother who was pleased to have a daughter:

She used to tell me she loved having a little girl, so that she could tell me all the secrets she wouldn't tell the boys or Dad. It was like a female conspiracy. I didn't like it as I got older, and I think she was very hurt by that.

For some, conflicting messages about success caused confusion and pain. Encouragement to do well at school was not always matched when success meant moving away from home:

I got a really good job when I was eighteen, but I had to move away from home. I felt I'd really let her down. And she told me I was getting too clever for my own good. That men don't want women who think they know it all.

Others remember being expected to help in the house, when the men of the family were all out playing football. One remembers being told: 'Don't sit there dreaming and reading, there's work to be done.' Her indignation was compounded by her brother and father both sitting behind newspapers at the time.

A common theme was that it is important to be a good mother and have a successful career, though many felt that the real pressure was somehow to resolve this conundrum, and manage both. A nurse in her late twenties with a young child described her mother saying:

Of course, I admire you. I mean. I couldn't have done it. I just couldn't have left you at that age. And your father wouldn't have allowed it. He supported us.

The various conflicting messages contained in that one statement are obvious.

Many of these mother–daughter relationships were described with considerable affection. They were not characterized by a lack of closeness, but by the daughters' real difficulty in establishing a separate identity, and handling conflicting demands and expectations. Although class and generation differences are to some extent apparent it is surprising, in talking to women, just how universal these themes are in mother–daughter relationships. It is also evident, as daughters themselves grow up, how they are able to recognize these themes in their own relationships with their own daughters. Even younger women, brought up in a household with a full-time working mother, and seen very much as persons in their own right, are still regarded as the primary carer, the nurturer, and the one who is always there.

Fathers and daughters

That less is written on father–daughter relationships than on those between mother and daughter is, perhaps, no surprise since it reflects reality. Mothers are generally present, fathers tend to come and go. This alone has enormous significance for the way girls come to understand female and male roles. Though the relationship with father is qualitatively significant, it is quantitively less in evidence. In our society, fathers occupy a somewhat paradoxical position; although actually absent from much of a child's day they are nevertheless experienced as both present and powerful. Whereas a mother's role is clear to the child, and directly experienced by her, the father occupies an external and largely incomprehensible world. Ursula Owen attempts to grasp this essential difference:

> In our culture mothering is a job, and fathering is a hobby. It may turn out to be a lifelong hobby but it is still a hobby. A father can choose his duties: there is no normal or essential behaviour that defines him. There is no such flexibility about mothering. The job is laid down, defined, set in cement. If mothers break the rules they are called to order, their status as mothers is questioned: for fathers there are no such clear rules to break.[11]

A young child is not able to comprehend anything beyond her actual experience. Time, space and distance, are all very immediate. Where father disappears to on a daily basis is at the same time mysterious, unattainable, yet also important. Boys, as they grow in the knowledge that they will be like their fathers, will come to recognize that they, too, will have entry into that other world. Girls receive a less clear message. Even if they have a mother who is working (most mothers of under-fives who work, do so, part-time) they are likely to be in the care of another woman, and mother still remains the primary carer. Women, out for an evening together, often refer to their partners as 'babysitting'. It is very rare for mothers to be described, or to describe themselves, in that way. Indeed, it would not make sense if they were; mothering is the essence of their role.

Girls learn from these early interactions with their father, that it is acceptable for men to come and go – indeed, it is essential and important that they do so. They learn that the person who will give them ongoing care and availability will be the mother. As a girl grows older, it is evident that her father can be very significant in facilitating, or otherwise, her ease of entry into a wider world. Ursula Owen suggests that:

> Some women have felt that fathers can make or break a daughter's confidence in her own power. The favoured daughter is often recognisable for her own confidence, her refusal to accept power-lessness.[12]

Perhaps this tells us that the power of the father, evident to the very small girl, can be used for or against her as she grows older. It is almost as if a daughter may only enter the male world with her father's permission. For many women this seems to extend to male partners later in life. That is, that they are part of a male world only on sufferance. They are allowed to be there. They are not there on merit, or fully in their own right.

As with memories of mothers, those of fathers are various, while also falling into some clear patterns. Many women remember their father as someone who was in some senses both special and important. Many remember being told to be good when he came in from work. Father would be tired. He had worked hard, and he was not to be bothered. Despite these injunctions, many had good memories of this being a special time of day. One woman recalls:

> I remember waiting for him by the gate, and tearing down the road towards him. He used to call me his little princess. When he was there he'd play with me, and talk to me. He was my special person. My mother was the everyday person. I still love seeing him.

Another says:

> My father made me believe in myself. He always encouraged me to think for myself, and to act for myself, and was there if it didn't work out. I carry him within me. I've always been able to have easy and trusting relationships with men and I'm sure that's why.

For others the power of their father was not so positive. The threat of 'wait until your father gets home,' was a real one for many, carrying with it apparent abdication of female authority. Another frequent recollection was of a mother who would not take any decision without consulting father. Some women remember feeling that their father was more interested in their brothers, and that they were excluded from male activities within, and without, the family. In a parallel way, some girls shared secrets with female family members, and remember the conspiracy of: 'we won't tell your Dad; men don't understand these things like women do'.

While some experience their fathers as deeply encouraging, others have the opposite experience:

I know I'm brighter than my brothers, and that I always have been. My father just would not allow that to be. He's always put me down, and if I've ever done well he dismisses it. He won't have anything to do with me now. I think he's willing me to fail, and then he'll talk to me again.

Another woman, abused by her father as a child, says:

It's affected my whole relationship with men. I either treat them as if they are helpless little boys who can't help themselves, and have to be looked after; or as if they are monsters who will destroy me. My father could smash me. Even when he's dead, I'll never be rid of him.

Many girls felt that their fathers liked them to look attractive, and remember being 'shown off' to friends and colleagues. They also became aware, as they grew older, that although father was powerful, he somehow also had to be looked after. His competence in the larger external world was apparently not matched by his ability to shop, unaided or unadvised, for clothes; to cook meals; or care for himself or others. Daughters, as they grew up, could be entrusted with these tasks, unlike male siblings, who often fell happily into the helpless male role.

A confusing picture emerges. Fathers – and, later, women's partners – tend to be seen in contradictory ways. They apparently have access to a world that is necessary for both status and economic survival, which gives them considerable power. That power can be expressed towards a daughter negatively or positively. She, too, may be encouraged into this world; or she may be actively discouraged. At the same time this important person is apparently helpless in everyday matters, and cannot manage without the level of help more obviously given to a child. Not only this, but he enters and exits from her life with not only impunity, but with positive approval. Mother, without such freedom, is the constant and caring figure, yet also portrayed as somehow less important. The daughter is prepared for being a woman and a mother, against this background of contradiction and paradox.

Girls: playing and being

Gender stereotyping arises not only in the central relationship at home. From a very young age a child also receives messages from the world which s/he sees outside the home. For instance, how does the world look to a three-year-old in the course of an everyday day? What part do men and women play in it? There are very few male nursery teachers, playgroup leaders or childminders. Most daytime groups cater for mothers and toddlers; fathers are a rarity. If the child is taken shopping, s/he will encounter predominantly female assistants. Men may be delivering things in lorries and they can be seen driving buses, delivering milk or emptying dustbins – they will be seen in essentially active roles, which to a small child seem quite exciting.

The women they see serve in shops, do the shopping and push other small children in prams and pushchairs – they will be essentially involved in being with others, caring for and serving them. They are more static, and more accessible. Milkmen, dustmen, and lorry drivers appear and disappear again, on their way to other places. During the course of the day, whether at home, at a childminder's or a nursery, meals will be cooked and presented by women, needs will be met by women, and any men in the picture are likely to be transitory. If they are taken to the park to play, they are likely to see other mothers or female carers with young children. Visits to a health clinic will reinforce this picture of a female world since most clinic helpers are women. So, for a small child, the immediate world is dominated by women. Men are around, but in the distance. They come and go, and are involved in more active and external pursuits. This continues through the early school years. Men have a very low presence in infant schools, and the first ongoing daily contact with a man for many girls will be a male teacher in junior school. It can be seen, then, that the world of a young child is very clearly defined in terms of gender-related role differentiation. As Sue Sharpe says:

> The active and passive dimensions of traditional male and female roles can be clearly seen in the way that a man's major activities are outward directed and a woman's are inner directed. He goes out to confront and capture the outside world while she constructs a cosy inside shelter for them both.[13]

We have already seen how clothing may restrict a girl's play. Studies[14] also show that girls and boys tend to be steered towards gender-specific toys, with the boys encouraged towards constructional toys and those demanding physical prowess. Another finding is that girls are more willing to play with boys' toys than boys are with girls'. This perhaps reflects the fact that it is more acceptable for a girl to be labelled a tomboy than it is for a boy to be a sissy. Whereas the former has some admirable connotations (and is well supported by some famous heroines in literature), and is labelled, at worst, as something girls grow out of, a sissy has no such positive associations. John and Elizabeth Newson point to the striking polarization of a child's play preference according to gender by the age of seven. Of girls' play at this age, they say:

> Girls' play tends to mirror fairly closely the role behaviour of those adult women who are constantly available to the children's observation in their daily lives: which means that it is concerned with looking after babies, keeping house, shopping, taking children to the doctor, and so on – all of which activities are very close to the real-life preoccupations of their own mothers, even where their own mother is at work.[15]

There is a considerable pressure for girls to be nurturing, responsible, and obedient, whereas boys are encouraged to be self-reliant and to be high achievers. Although this appears to be true across cultures, there are also important class differences within cultures. Sue Sharpe argues that 'working class girls are likely to become more immediately aware of the different expectations and roles of men and women'.[16] Such pressure, reinforced by girls' view of the world, has considerable effect on how they see themselves, and how they are able to play and to be.

Education and careers

Nowadays, all subjects are supposed to be open to all children. Gone are the days of cookery just for girls and woodwork just for boys. Yet, at the age when choices are made, girls still veer towards arts subjects, and boys towards sciences. In view of earlier life experiences, this will come as no surprise. Girls choose different subjects, and are then, as adults, underrepresented in senior positions throughout society. So what is happening to girls?

In the early school years the acquisition of reading skills is a key area. Analysis of reading schemes used in schools shows that girls and women are underrepresented, and stereotypically portrayed. Loban,[17] examining six reading schemes, found that only three adult female roles were presented – mother, grandmother and aunt. By contrast, thirteen adult male roles were presented, including builder, postman and shop owner. Girls were seen participating in only three activities: preparing tea, playing with dolls, and taking care of younger siblings. Boys were involved in a wider range of seven activities, including playing with cars, trains, footballs and gardening.

In another study by Frazier *et al.*[18] it is suggested that troublesome boys received the most time and attention, and that quiet and well-behaved girls, encouraged in that way of behaving, received little. Sue Sharpe comments that:

> In fact, the quietness, obedience and passivity of girls is often held up as a mark of their greater maturity and responsibility. It is ironic that these same attitudes are later used to demonstrate inferiority.[19]

Working-class girls, more likely to be both troublesome in the classroom and disillusioned with school, are the most likely to leave as soon as possible, and enter low-status jobs. Grazyna Baran points out that:

> Girls, especially working-class and immigrant girls, lack confidence in themselves and their abilities, especially in unfamiliar areas. Girls exert pressures on each other which reinforce this lack of confidence. There is a pressure not to brag, show yourself up or make a fuss; otherwise you may be labelled big-headed. Discretion and modesty are valued, while outspokenness and self-assertion are suspect.[20]

Dale Spender has analysed the amount of time teachers give to girl pupils, compared to the time given to boys. She convincingly concludes that boys are both responded to more quickly, otherwise they become disruptive, and given a higher proportion of teacher time. This occurred even when teachers had been instructed to share their time equally between boys and girls, and believed that they were doing so:

> 'I was so conscious of trying to spend more time with the girls that I really thought I had overdone it' one teacher said in amazement when she listened to the evidence of the tape and worked out that in her interactions with the students only 36 per cent of her time had been spent with girls. 'But I thought I spent more time with the girls' said another who found she had given them 34 per cent of her attention, 'and', she added, 'the boys thought so too. They were complaining about me talking to the girls all the time.'[21]

Girls who do continue through the education system rarely

reach the same level as do their male peers. Not only do they receive less attention, but women of all ages recall messages given to them at school, and the influence of these on them. One, a care assistant in her fifties, recalls:

> If you were a girl and you'd failed the eleven plus, you'd had it. You may work for a year or two, but really what you'd do was get married and have kids. That's what you were educated for. And they [teachers] were more interested in the boys.

A teacher in her forties remembers:

> I was strongly advised against even thinking about medicine, which I was really interested in. I was steered firmly towards teaching. I was quite explicitly told that it would fit in better with a husband and children. That it would be easy to return to when they were older. And I was only seventeen, or eighteen. I was also told that men don't like women to be too clever. That they like to be the boss.

A young woman in her twenties, educated in a mixed comprehensive, says that:

> You could choose to do the traditional boys' subjects, and I think a lot of teachers would have supported you. But you had to be quite brave, and some girls were, because you could feel really lonely and different, and you could get teased.

Certainly, to break into traditional male realms requires a degree of self-confidence and self-belief that girls are not generally brought up to possess. An eighteen-year-old girl, the only one in her year on an engineering course, expressed this:

> Walking in that room on the first day was hell. They all stopped talking, and its been very lonely. And I always feel I must do really well, and if I don't, everyone knows immediately. I can't hide, as the only girl I'm always noticed.

Girls are often ambivalent towards academic success.[22] Studies show that both sexes envisage unpleasant futures for the successful and clever woman. However, both sexes are equally positive about the futures of men who are successful. Girls and women may have to walk a thin line between doing well and doing too well. The message of 'now don't you try to be *too* clever' is one that has been heard by many. In career terms, the dilemma is often that of having to be especially good to get a job and, once in it, not so good that male colleagues are threatened. In addition to all these pressures, an outstanding one for so many women, often envisaged by them in girlhood, is how to be both a mother and a worker. It is, perhaps, surprising just how many women achieve so much. How much more, one wonders, might they achieve if they were more actively encouraged?

Sexuality

Women of different ages and generations may be expected to have received greatly varying views and messages on the subject of sexuality. The adolescence, half a century ago, of women now in their sixties and seventies was a very different time from that of women brought up since the availability of the pill and abortion. Nowadays, sex need not lead to conception. Women have won some control over their bodies. It is assumed nowadays that girls and young women will readily and easily acquire information about their bodies and sex, and that this, combined with the less judgemental attitudes of recent years, will leave them free to express and explore their sexuality.

While it is true that availability of contraception has made an enormous difference in the lives of women, it should not be assumed that this has eradicated other difficulties. Sex certainly takes on a high profile in today's world, but this does not mean that sexuality is a straightforward issue for women. On the one hand, they may now be told that they have a right to enjoy sex; on the other, they are surrounded by images of women being portrayed as sexual objects, there for the enjoyment of men. John Berger describes how women are turned into objects:

> *men act* and *women appear*. Men look at women. Women watch themselves being looked at. This determines not only most relations between men and women, but also the relation of women to themselves. The surveyor of woman in herself is male: the surveyed female. Thus she turns herself into an object – and most particularly an object of vision: a sight.[23]

It should also not be assumed that accurate sexual knowledge has necessarily accompanied a more liberal atmosphere. The assumption that today's children know it all is not borne out by the experience of many. As Carol Lee states:

> Because teenagers have developed their own aggressive way of expressing their feelings about sex and because advertisers have an equally aggressive interest in the subject, we imagine that sex has become mentionable. This is not so. In eight years of meeting

parents, teachers and pupils and in discussing the subject with other
sex educators, all my experience has borne out the fact that, except
in the most cursory of terms, sex is still unmentionable.[24]

While sexuality and sexual activity may be far more explicitly
portrayed, and whilst more is written and discussed, this is not
necessarily reflected in accurate information reaching young girls,
or in sensible and honest discussion. For many, as they enter
adolescence, awareness of themselves as sexual beings is accompanied by warnings of the potential dangers of this. The risk of
rape, and other forms of sexual abuse and harassment, is very
much in evidence for the modern young woman trying to make
and take her own place in the world. At the same time, women are
aware, through advertising, media influence, and peer-group
pressure, of the importance of looking attractive.

Women themselves can remember vividly the mixed and
confusing messages about sex passed on to them by parents,
teachers and others in their adolescent years. One woman in her
sixties remembers being told:

> Men like it, and women don't, but you have to put up with it or else
> they'll find someone else.

This 'lie back and think of England' approach to sexual relationships appears to be common in women's recollections. They often
report being given no hard facts, and what exactly 'it' was
supposed to be was hazy in the extreme. Nevertheless, it was a
woman's duty to respond, and to put up with her partner's
inability to contain his sexual desires; these had to be met. The
woman quoted above encountered another complication: she did
enjoy sex and felt, as a young married woman, abnormal and
guilty.

Other women report being told that 'nice girls don't', but that
'it's better to marry a man who knows what he's doing'. (Who
teaches them in the first place, one wonders? Not, presumably, a
nice girl!) Other common messages women remember are the
following:

> Men don't want second-hand goods.
>
> Always look good; take pride in your appearance; but don't tease.
>
> You're asking for it if you go out dressed like that.
>
> Always have your make up on, your hair done, and the children and
> the house tidy when he comes home. He won't want to see a mess at
> the end of a long day.

Watch your figure and don't let yourself go.

It's not safe to be out by yourself at night. Always carry an alarm, and avoid direct eye contact with men. Watch and listen carefully.

At the core of all these well-remembered sayings is a universal experience of women's bodies and sexuality as existing primarily for men's enjoyment. This is accompanied by the warning that being a woman is dangerous, and exposes you to the possibility of sexual attack. As a result of this, it is women who must exercise vigilance. After all, men cannot help it. However much women challenge this view of their sexuality – and, of course, many do – it seems as if a long struggle lies ahead before fundamental and lasting change occurs. It should also be remembered that while heterosexual women struggle with these issues, the situation for lesbian women is even more fraught. They encounter further layers of oppression and uninformed predujice, as they define their sexuality not in terms of pleasing men, but of pleasing themselves and another within a female relationship.

Relating and relationships

From early on in a girl's life it is evident that much of her being revolves around her relatedness with others. As has already been shown, this is reflected in the way she plays as a small child, and it is further demonstrated in how she envisages her future as she enters adolescence. Talking to teachers, it is evident that working-class girls in particular see their future as centred around partner and children, whereas middle-class girls, more likely to have mothers in professional jobs, see wider horizons. Sue Sharpe notes that:

> Boyfriends feature heavily in the thoughts and activities of teenage girls whether or not they have actually got one. They represent social success and status, a secure symbol of acceptable femininity.[25]

Three-quarters of the girls in her study wanted to be married by the time they were twenty-five, and a similar result is shown in a study of first-year students.[26] Women students were asked to look at their options fifteen years on, and very few saw themselves as either single or childless. About half wanted to be married, with children, and having a career. Liz Heron also feels that:

Home, marriage, motherhood come to enter the picture of imagined futures increasingly with adolescence, even if the dominant scenario in the foreground is something else: a job, career, travel.[27]

Very few young women envisage a future without a partner. Life without a man is not part of the package deal on offer in Western society. The fact that many women do successfully and happily live alone is given little cognizance or encouragement. The myth and the facts do not add up. Women are brought up with the vague expectation of secure male support, the knowledge of male power, and the unacceptability of their own independence and assertiveness. This denial of female independence, and encouragement towards dependency, at once reduces and invalidates women, and steers round the issue of male dependency:

> Women's economic dependence on men has been a perennial smokescreen for male dependence. It confirms the view of women as weak and men as strong, women as needy and men as providers. It hides the solid bedrock of female emotional strength, shoring up the male edifice of self-sufficiency.[28]

A young woman of twenty describes the conflict for her between an independent lifestyle, and settling down:

> Part of me wants to rush off and do exciting things, and not even think about marriage or kids. My brother spent a couple of years travelling around and really enjoyed it. My friend and I thought about doing that, but my parents say they'd never have a moment's peace until I was safe back. My boyfriend wants us to get married and says he can't be expected to wait while I go off enjoying myself. The trouble is, I see marriage as a bit of an insurance policy: it would be safe and protect me.

It is also evident from being with, and working with, women, how much pleasure they take in being women. They often delight in the closeness they experience with female friends; value enormously their role as mothers; and experience a richness in being that they sense is rarely felt by men. They may feel that men have, in some respects, a more straightforward life; they may resent the restrictions on opportunities for women, and feel they can carry too much of too many burdens. Still, against the odds it may seem, they like being women. Men may have power and influence, but they do not want to be like them, or to be men. Women, in my experience, are not envious of men, although they may well resent their power.

Implications for counselling women

I suggested at the beginning of this chapter that in order to make sense of issues women bring to therapy and counselling, it is necessary to have some understanding of the processes and events that bring them to womanhood. The next chapter looks specifically at some of the gender issues that can arise in therapy, but the following are some illustrations of how the points already raised affect the lives of women, and the situations they bring to their counsellor or therapist. What is common to them, and is often evident among women clients, is their rapid descent into guilt, responsibility, anxiety, low self-esteem and self-blame. In today's society, the cult of the individual makes it all too easy for women to fall into the pit of self-blame; it has almost become a virtue to do so. In this context it is crucial that those who work with women are aware both of the impact of gender stereotyping and of the effect of the second-class-citizen label. These examples show us that we need to understand that the source of an individual's guilt, anxiety or depression, does not spring solely from the individual psyche. It must be recognized, and taken into account, that another source arises from the way society is organized. Recognizing both levels as significant, allows exploration of both internal and external worlds, acknowledging the power and respective influence of both. This enables and encourages the uniqueness of the individual, while at the same time telling her she is not alone. In this way, her empowerment is encouraged; self-confidence can begin to be built, and choices and possibilities identified.

Claire, aged nineteen, was raped by a friend after she had allowed him to stay the night. He had stayed before; and in her circle of friends this was a fairly usual occurrence. As far as she was concerned, he was a friend; on this occasion he would sleep on her floor as previously. There was no problem. She 'couldn't believe it' when he demanded to have intercourse with her. She refused; he forced her to have sex, and then left. As a result of this she became pregnant:

> The consultant didn't believe me when I said I'd been raped and I heard him say to the registrar 'What did she expect to happen, having him in the room with her. Of course she wasn't raped.' His examination of me was awful; it was like being raped again. I feel it was all my fault. I feel eaten up with guilt. That I just asked for it. I feel ashamed and bad and dirty.

Jill, aged thirty, has a senior management post. Her partner of nine years has left her, and married a woman of twenty-one:

> He always said he wanted an equal relationship, but in the end he didn't. When I started to earn more than him, he just didn't want to know. He wanted me to stay at home and have a baby really, and I couldn't stand that. I don't know who I am any more. Why do I feel so panicky? Why do I think I just can't survive alone? But I do. And I just feel it's impossible to be in a relationship and to be me. I feel hopeless.

Carol, aged twenty-five, has four children between one and nine years. She was abused by her father as a child, and is now regularly attacked by her partner. She has no money, no job, and has recently returned to her partner, having left accommodation found for her by a women's refuge:

> Well, you know what they're like don't you. I mean they're all the same, just like my Dad, can't help themselves. They're children really, aren't they. You just have to watch out when they've had a few; you know, keep them happy like. And I can't manage by myself – my Mum and Dad have always said I can't look after myself. I get lonely you see. After all, you're not much without a man are you?

Notes

1   Sharpe, S. (1976). *'Just Like a Girl'*. Penguin, p. 62.
2   Chodorow, N. (1978). *The Reproduction of Mothering*. University of California Press.
3   Oakley, A. (1979). *Becoming a Mother*. Martin Robertson.
4   Moss, H.A. (1967). 'Sex, age, and state as determinants of mother–infant interaction', *Merrill Palmer Quarterly*. 13, pp. 19–36.
5   Hartley, R. (1966). 'A Developmental View of Female Sex-Role Identification' in Biddle, J. and Thomas E.J. (eds), *Role Theory*. John Wiley.
6   Grabucker, M. (1988). *There's a Good Girl*. The Women's Press, p. 7.
7   Ibid., p. 162.
8   Chodorow, *The Reproduction of Mothering*, p. 109.
9   Dinnerstein, D. (1987). *The Rocking of the Cradle and the Ruling of the World*. The Women's Press, p. 81.
10   Ibid., p. 94.
11   Owen, U. (ed.) (1983). *Father's: Reflections by Daughters*. Virago, p. 13.
12   Ibid., p. 13.
13   Sharpe, *'Just Like a Girl'*, p. 68.

14 Hartup, W. (1963). 'Avoidance of inappropriate sex typing by young children', *Journal of Consulting Psychology*, 27; Wolf, T. (1973). 'Effects of live modelled sex-inappropriate behaviour in a naturalistic setting', *Developmental Psychology*, 9.

15 Newson, E. and Newson, J. (1976). *Seven Years Old in the Home Environment*. George Allen & Unwin, p. 157.

16 Sharpe, '*Just Like a Girl*', p. 72.

17 Loban, G. (1976). *Sex Roles in Reading Schemes*. Children's Rights Workshop.

18 Frazier, N. and Sadler, M. (1973). *Sexism in School and Society*. Harper and Row.

19 Sharpe, '*Just Like a Girl*', p. 146.

20 Baran, G. (1987), 'Teaching Girls Science', in McNeil, M. (ed.), *Gender and Expertise*. Free Assciation Books, p. 91.

21 Spender, D. (1989). *Invisible Women*. The Women's Press, p. 56.

22 Monahan, L. *et al.* (1974). 'Intraphysic versus cultural explanations of the fear of success motives', *Journal of Personality and Social Psychology*, 29.

23 Berger, J. (1972). *Ways of Seeing*. Penguin, p. 47 (emphasis in original).

24 Lee, C. (1983). *The Ostrich Position*. Writers and Readers Co-op., p. 1.

25 Sharpe, '*Just Like a Girl*', p. 214.

26 Epstein, G. and Bronzaft, A. (1972). 'Female freshmen view their roles as women', *Journal of Marriage and the Family*, 34.

27 Heron, L. (1986). *Changes of Heart*. Pandora Press, p. 34.

28 Ibid., p. 109.

4

Gender, mental health and counselling

She had remained sure that somewhere in what they called a
hospital was someone who cared for you, someone with
answers, someone who could tell her what was wrong with
her and mold her to a better life. But the pressure was to say
please and put on lipstick and sit at a table playing cards, to beg
and work for nothing, cleaning the houses of the staff. To look
away from graft and abuse. To keep quiet as you watched them
beat other patients. To pretend that the rape in the linen room
was a patient's fantasy.

Marge Piercy

First encounters sometimes tell us little, sometimes a lot. Conversation may be superficial or it may lead to the exchange of
confidences. But two things which are always immediately
evident are the gender and colour of the person encountered. Age
may also be a factor, but this is a much broader category, and
nowadays less clearly defined by external appearance, such as
style of dress. Age we may mistake; class can be uncertain, while
gender and race stare us in the face. Assumptions and stereotypes
abound about both, and, as we have seen in the previous chapter,
gender issues are wide-ranging and deep-seated. Statements such
as: 'We don't notice she's a girl any more', 'She's just one of the
lads', or 'He's my best friend, it doesn't matter that he's black',
contain both truths and falsehoods. The message that is intended,
and is communicated, is that the relationship is close enough not
to be overwhelmed by gender or race, which ceases to be an
immediate focus. It is the whole person who is seen. What a person
is like within is of more value than externals. The very wording of
these statements indicates that however much the relationship
and the person are valued, attention still needs to be drawn to
whether the person is a man or woman, boy or girl, black or white.
This remains so even when the object of the statement is to
express the opposite, and when that person is genuinely appreciated in his/her own right. Indeed, for most of us, the fact of our

colour and gender is central to our identity and being. It may, or may not, cause us difficulties, but we would not want it lost or obscured.

The immediate visibility of gender is obvious. Its ongoing significance may be of a more complex nature, and what is apparently external also lies at the core of the person. The degree and extent to which gender affects so many aspects of a woman's life is largely hidden from public gaze – inevitably, perhaps, when so much of her life is engaged in highly personalized activities. As the last two chapters have indicated, as the personal becomes more public, a picture of discrimination and limited opportunity is evident. It is important to ask whether women's treatment in the mental health services maintains the status quo, reinforcing stereotypes, and encouraging the acceptance of the unacceptable. Does it place unfair emphasis on the individual rather than tackle underlying structural and political issues? Taking therapy and counselling, is it a means whereby liberal-minded individuals can earn a living that is a reasonable sop to their consciences, in a country like the UK, where more radical political activity seems a non-starter in present times? Do therapists and counsellors, in their work with women, really acknowledge the complexities of their lives, and the impact of gender issues both generally and within the therapeutic relationship? How do they incorporate awareness into their work?

The quick answer is that some counsellors and therapists are blissfully unaware that such issues even exist. This lack of awareness may be blissful for the counsellor, though not for the client. The ability of the counsellor to think one-dimensionally, as if only straight lines existed, is a comfortable way of being. It is not helpful for clients who themselves are caught up in experiences of tortuous complexity, and for whom straight lines have disappeared a long time ago. Other counsellors are aware of the issues, but think themselves immune from falling into stereotypical traps. George Stricker[1] suggests that because the therapist concentrates on the individual, sex stereotyping is somehow avoided. This is the therapeutic equivalent to the ostrich approach: if you maneouvre into a position where something is out of view, it ceases to exist. In this way realities go unseen. They are neither confronted nor acknowledged. Central aspects of women's lives are avoided.

Another approach is reflected in the growth of feminist therapy, women's therapy centres, and other counselling services

run by women for women. These represent an active acknowledgement of women's lives as a whole. They have a political as
well as a psychological awareness, and work within the context of
both. However, it is sometimes argued that a political and feminist
stance clashes with a therapeutic approach, and that the former
invalidates the latter. Dorothy Tennov expresses this view:

> But if the feminist who wishes to engage in psychotherapy uses the
> trappings of psychodynamic theory, is she not misleading her
> potential clients? If she now interprets her clients' behaviour is she
> now engaging in oppressive and abusive actions?[2]

It should be said that feminist therapists and counsellors represent
a wide range of theoretical backgrounds. Those who incorporate a
psychodynamic framework feel that social structures and external
realities certainly influence the internal world of an individual.
They also believe in an interrelatedness between the two, and
constantly attempt in their work with women to maintain that
awareness.

There is perhaps another group of counsellors and therapists
who have some theoretical knowledge of gender issues but have
not as yet translated the theory into practice. Unlike those who
take the ostrich approach, they do not actually bury their heads in
the sand, but they develop a nice line in looking the other way
while pretending not to. It is evident, for example, that many of
those who train counsellors and therapists will acknowledge the
centrality of gender issues. Far fewer actually incorporate this into
their course structures. Gender issues, and awareness of their
significance, should be interwoven into the basic fabric of course
material. They should not be added as an afterthought, as is often
the case.

It is important to remember that most clients of all mental
health services are women. These services fail to recognize the
complex issues of being a woman in society, and the effect on their
mental health. This is another aspect of their oppression. It is only
in recent years that there have been moves to understand the
psychology of women in their own right, carrying with it the
recognition of the need to create a framework that is not saturated
in male terms, expectations and definitions.

Appreciation of gender issues in couselling women not only
requires understanding how girls and women are brought up
but also how psychiatric and other mental health services respond
to them. The philosophy of those who are currently concerned

with providing services run by women for women, and those who would categorize themselves as feminist therapists, arises out of a dissatisfaction and dislike at the way they see women being treated.

How have they reached that position? In order to answer this question we need to ask a further question: how have women been treated within our mental health, medical and other services when they experience difficulties? Answering that, we find a perspective for examining feminist therapy, and for considering the implications of whether women clients should be seen by male or female therapists and counsellors.

Women and the psychiatric and medical services

Although the 1970s and 1980s saw an increase in the availability of specific and separate counselling and therapy services for women, many are still treated within the framework of psychiatric facilities or by general practitioners. In the history and development of psychiatry, women are under-represented as senior policy-making staff, though over-represented as patients. The position may now be changing somewhat, but women have historically been excluded from active and influential participation in the medical and psychiatric professions, as they have been from all others. Once more, the male voice has dominated, and that of women has not been heard.

The misuse of benzodiazepines (minor tranquillizers) in 'treating' women, and the resulting agonies this has caused for many, are now acknowledged. Although there is now greater awareness of the dangers of over prescribing these drugs, they were once seen as a panacea for many of the problems experienced by women and identified as psychologically caused. Joy Melville[3] describes how, in one year, out of 115 advertisements for tranquillizers, hypnotics, and anti-depressants in the *British Medical Journal*, ninety-one identified women as the patients. At the time of writing her book, out of 21 million people taking tranquillizers or sedatives in Britain 14 million were women. Being sedate and tranquil have traditionally been viewed as desirable feminine attributes. Perhaps this extraordinarily high level of prescribing reflects society's desire to maintain women in this quiet role. It is easier than uncovering the variety of social ills that lie beneath the symptoms. This is reflected in a study carried out by Gayford,[4] who discovered that out of 100 battered wives, nearly three-quarters had been prescribed either tranquillizers or anti-depressants. In another study women are shown to be the main candidates for other drugs, too:

> Women have now become the primary clientele for psychotropic drugs; in the late 1970s studies showed that 21 per cent of the women in the patient population, as compared to 9.7 per cent of the men, received such medication.[5]

Whether such prescribing is appropriate, or whether, as I suggest, it reflects other factors in operation, is, of course, a very important question, and many of those who work with women do not believe it is being adequately or seriously addressed. Is such a difference in the prescribing rates really justified, and actually helpful? Or could it be that the male-dominated profession does not understand what lies behind the manifestation of symptoms (as indicated in Gayford's study) and is dealing with these in isolation, rather than within their context? Further, are such symptoms understood differently if they are exhibited by men? Might some symptoms or behaviours quite simply be more acceptable in men than in women? What in men is likely to be seen as normal can often be interpreted as a sign of mental illness in women. No wonder, then, that such symptoms do not readily respond to drugs.

Some studies convincingly give support to the truth of this argument, notably one carried out by Inge Broverman and her colleagues. They examined the sex role stereotypes of a group of mental health professionals, asking them to define mentally healthy men, women and adults. The characteristics ascribed to the mentally healthy adult corresponded very closely to the description of the healthy man. Not so for women: 'clinicians are significantly less likely to attribute traits that characterise healthy adults to a woman than they are likely to attribute these traits to a healthy man'. In other words, what is seen as normal for a woman does not match up with what is seen as normal for an adult. Inge Broverman describes how:

> clinicians are more likely to suggest that healthy women differ from healthy men by being more submissive; less independent; less adventurous; more easily influenced; less aggressive; less competitive; more excitable in minor crises; having their feelings more easily hurt; being more emotional; more concerned about their appearance; less objective; and disliking maths and science. This constellation seems a most unusual way of describing any mature, healthy individual.[6]

It can be seen from this that women can be labelled ill, disturbed or neurotic if they display characteristics that are not perceived as mentally healthy; whereas in a man the same characteristics are seen as healthy. This is further supported by the clinical experience of practitioners. Certain behaviours exhibited by women are seen as unacceptable, and are more likely to be labelled as symptoms of disturbance that require 'treatment'. The following examples illustrate the point:

A therapist, in his work with a woman with a history of abuse in childhood had been encouraging her to acknowledge and express the anger that seemed locked inside her and that interfered with many aspects of her life. One night, a row developed between her and her husband. Unusually, instead of becoming frightened, withdrawn and depressed, she stood her ground, asserted her viewpoint and when this was ignored by her husband, became angry. In the context of the argument, her response appeared appropriate, and certainly understandable. Both she and her husband started drinking; she became angrier, threw a bottle across the room (nowhere near her husband) and it smashed. Her husband rang the family doctor, saying that his wife had gone completely crazy. The more she protested, the more her husband's view became reinforced. The doctor visited, called out another colleague, and the situation escalated. Admission to psychiatric hospital was considered but finally rejected. The woman concerned was told she must 'calm down'; her husband agreed that he could cope if she 'behaved herself'. Throughout this (and this was verified by the two male professionals involved), no one talked with her about why she was angry, either in terms of the immediate situation or her past history.

The implications of this incident were considerable: the damage done to the therapeutic relationship was huge; she was treated in a way that reflected her own earlier abuse – she was not listened to, and her experiences were invalidated. Additionally, it was clearly and forcefully indicated that the expression of anger was unacceptable; that it would show she was 'crazy', and that, ultimately, unless contained, could result in admission to psychiatric hospital against her wishes. But we have to ask: would a man who became angry and drunk, and smashed a bottle, be treated in this way? The answer, I suspect, is 'no'.

A psychiatric nurse described working with an Asian woman, who had been admitted to her ward and spoke little English. The nurse felt that her agitation, and her angry manner, were a result of fear and frustration. She was unable to communicate freely and easily; she found herself in an alien world; her home situation was highly problematic; and she was worried about her children. Because of the language difficulty, she required time and patience which many of the staff were unable or unwilling to give. The non-availability of either an interpreter, or a member of staff speaking the same language, in a major hospital of a multi-cultural city seems highly unacceptable in itself. But added to this, when the nurse attempted to explain the woman's behaviour as she understood it – response to a frightening situation – she found that she, too, was not listened to. When she persisted, the psychiatrist suggested that she was becoming over-involved. He diagnosed the patient as having a psychotic disorder and prescribed drugs accordingly. In this way, not only were the circumstances and complex life experiences of the patient ignored and invalidated, but so also were the skills and sensitivity of a nurse with considerable expertise. Both were made powerless, and the nurse was left disillusioned, wondering if there was any point in trying to be assertive on behalf of patients. She recognized that she was in danger of being labelled as both difficult and emotionally over-involved. She also knew that once she was perceived in this way, the chances of ever being listened to were slight. Both female clients and staff can effectively be rendered invisible and powerless by such means.

A social worker had been working for some time with a single mother who was struggling to re-establish herself after a period of depression. She had received psychiatric treatment, although the social worker felt the depression was in fact a response to a very difficult life situation. She was in her thirties, with a young daughter. The daughter was experiencing difficulties at school, and during a case discussion with the various professionals involved, it was suggested by one that the child's difficulties were a response to all the different men in her mother's life. When the social worker questioned the facts behind the judgement, it transpired that her client had only ever had two relationships, and that both men had been known to the child and apparently accepted. Behind such a suggestion seemed to be a value-loaded assumption, that women, especially mothers, have no right to a sexual life. The dual morality that happily allows men to behave in a particular way while heaping disapproval on women who act similarly, is still very much in evidence. In this instance, the social worker pointed out that in the same circumstances, a single father would be likely to be praised for his efforts, and, she believed, his sexual life would not even have been seen as relevant. It transpired that the child's difficulties arose from a problem, easily resolvable, at school. That may not have become apparent if the social worker had not been confident enough to challenge the initial incorrect assumption.

A woman in her forties, severely depressed and experiencing strong suicidal feelings, described the time, ten years previously, when she had been admitted to a psychiatric hospital following a large overdose. Her marriage had been an unhappy one, and her husband's violence, towards both her and their children, so great that she had feared for her life. Following her admission, a 'history' of her life was taken from her husband. Not surprisingly, he did not mention the violence. When, eventually, she was seen by the same doctor, he told her how lucky she was to have such a supportive husband. He also told her not to worry about the children; her husband had arranged time off work to care for them. He did not check the husband's story with her. Indeed, he made no attempt to ascertain the facts as she saw them. He assumed the husband's story to be correct, and, on the basis of this wrong assumption, a detailed treatment plan was formulated. She felt she had been labelled as ill; that she would, therefore, not be believed; that any attempt at explanation would simply increase the danger in the situation for her and the children, and would further reinforce the view of her as unstable. The opportunity to work with her was not used. Ten years later her difficulties had become firmly entrenched, and her distrust of anyone in the caring professions was extreme.

There have been some attempts to create alternative models of psychiatric care, incorporating a different analysis both of society and of a person's symptoms. The anti-psychiatry movement of the 1960s held considerable promise, but appears to have evaporated since then. However, R.D. Laing's work, particularly his publication, with Aaron Esterson, of *Sanity, Madness and the Family*[7] had considerable impact at the time. The book argued, with some force, that symptoms displayed by women, and identified as madness, were attempts both to make sense of a senseless situation, and to deal with contradictory demands, often implied but rarely made explicit. In this way, dealing with them directly or explicitly was made impossible. One way through this was for women to develop apparently senseless or bizarre actions or words. Laing and Esterson argued that when examined in the context of the situation women were in, and when they were listened to, the apparently senseless made sense. The work of David Cooper[8] and Joseph Burke,[9] was also influential at this time, and two books by Irving Goffman[10] added more weight to this radical understanding of mental illness.

Talking with recent consumers of mental health services, it seems that these ideas, developed in the 1960s, have largely become submerged. What is noticeable is how little the women who use these services are consulted about what would actually help them. Some changes have, of course, occurred. Long-stay admissions to psychiatric hospitals have generally ceased. The emphasis is on care in the community, although without sufficient resources to allow this to become a reality. Much remains the same. Apart from occasional pockets of excellence, there is a general lack of awareness of issues affecting women, although they remain the majority of users of the service. It is worth remembering how male-dominated the medical profession is: in 1985, 84.5 per cent of nurses and 20 per cent of general practitioners were women. In 1986 86.4 per cent of consultants and senior hospital medical officers were men.[11]

It is evident that psychiatry largely ignores, or even refuses to see, issues of gender as relevant in its treatment of women. Perhaps those responsible for training in medicine and in psychiatry need to ask themselves why such an important area has for so long been ignored. But many other professions are involved in working with women, often in a setting that they describe as counselling. Are they any more aware of these issues?

The caring professions

Apart from medicine, perhaps the two other professional groups most obviously involved in working with women are social workers and psychologists. Social work, in particular, is female-dominated at a practice level, and male-dominated at a senior management level. It is perhaps difficult to assess the effect on women clients of a situation where the worker assigned to them is not the one who can take decisions when there are policy or resource implications involved. There may, for instance, be a policy that allows short-term work only, or that decides which clients are going to receive priority. These decisions are likely to be taken at a senior management level. The degree to which social workers are consulted will vary between authorities. In the final analysis it is a management decision, in which women's interests are likely to be underrepresented. So women clients, representing those with least power in society, are seen by women who, in organizational and political terms, frequently have little control over what they can offer.

Many social work training courses nowadays place an emphasis on encouraging awareness of issues of both gender and race. In this respect social workers seem to be ahead of their colleagues in psychology; certainly some clinical psychology training courses almost totally ignore these aspects of the person. However thorough the latter's training is in other respects, questions remain about the overall effectiveness of such training when central questions like these are not given prominence. Individual psychology has to be translated into effective practice, which cannot happen if gender barriers have not been acknowledged. The individual woman needs to be seen as part of a wider world. It is important that recent, and challenging, literature on women's psychology comes to occupy a major place in course material. The work of such authors as Dorothy Dinnerstein,[12] Juliet Mitchell,[13] Jean Baker Miller,[14] Nancy Chodorow,[15] and Susie Orbach and Luise Eichenbaum[16] is enormously significant in the ongoing and developing debate on women's issues.

Gender issues can be clearly seen in the work of those in the caring professions, and again case examples illustrate this most clearly:

A male psychologist had been seeing a new female client for a few weeks. He described his client as having been sexually abused by her father and uncle. He felt he had a good working relationship with her. She was able to be very open with him, and had been quite happy to see a man. However, he began to feel that no progress was being made, although she showed no outward signs of unfriendliness towards him. When the psychologist's supervisor suggested that perhaps seeing a man was problematic for her, the psychologist at first rejected this; he had been careful to ascertain her feelings on this. He was even somewhat reproachful to his supervisor for making such a suggestion. However, when this was considered further, and connected to the impossibility of the client's ever being able to say no to her father and uncle, the suggestion made more sense. In addition, what he had not considered at all was her overall position of powerlessness in terms of her present-day position.

She was a young woman, in a poorly paid job, where all the

women were in very subservient positions to the men. It was non-
unionized; jobs could be lost easily, and she saw no hope of
anything better or different. For her, saying 'no' to any man about
anything was quite inconceivable. His initial discussion with her,
although well intentioned, had been an absolute non-starter. It
had no meaning to her. Her inability to say 'no' had a long history.
Her father and her uncle had ignored such a response; indeed, it
led to worse abuse. It seemed that her apparent openness with the
psychologist had been a similar reaction: 'It's best to give a man
what he wants, or he'll do worse things to you, and make you
suffer more.' Her experiences in the world as an adolescent and
young woman had reinforced her feeling of lack of power. This
central issue became the focus of work with her. It could not be
dealt with by an enquiry in the first session and put away thereafter. It was not until the psychologist himself understood both
levels of her experience – the personal and the structural – and
their considerable effect, that he was able to start helping his client
explore them and understand them for herself. In doing so, she
became freer to make choices for herself. For instance, she decided
to try for a place on a 'fresh start' scheme at the local college, and
this represented a major move for her.

An example of gender stereotyping that is not uncommon is
provided by a psychologist who was seeing a woman who lived
with her mother. In a tone of some surprise, he remarked on how
efficiently they managed, and how well they kept the house. The
stereotype that a woman cannot possibly manage without a man is
a popular one. All the evidence to the contrary is conveniently
ignored. Perhaps the underlying fear for men is that women
actually manage very well without them. And where does that
leave men? When male professionals, already in a position of
power, communicate their belief in this stereotype to their women
clients, it is harmful, invalidating and patronizing. Many men
seem to communicate just this kind of attitude without, apparently, knowing that they are doing so. Men who are consciously
sexist can be responded to rather more easily; unconscious sexism
is more problematic, particularly when the man in question
believes himself not to be so.

The stereotype can operate in reverse. A social worker described
how one of her clients, a male single parent, managed to hold down
a job and look after his two school-age children. She was most
admiring of his abilities, and gave him considerable support, as did
the firm he worked for. She was able to recognize that she did not

describe single mothers she knew in a similar way. None of them received concessions from their workplace, and they certainly did not receive such an accolade. Again, if that attitude was communicated to her clients it could be very demoralizing to women already struggling. It suggests that a man who manages to do a difficult job, is much more valued, because he has more inherent value, than a woman in the same situation.

A final example was reported by an experienced social worker. She had been working with a woman who was very depressed. Her living conditions were appalling and the social worker had battled with various agencies in order to get more assistance. In this she had not succeeded. Her client had said to her that she was not to worry; she had done her best. She added that really, the social worker was in just the same position as her. They were both women, and neither of them could do anything about anything. It was just the way the world was. She did wonder, however, if it would have made any difference if the social worker's male boss had seen her instead. The difficulty for the social worker was that she was wondering the same thing. It can sometimes be easy for women helpers to fall into a state of mutual depression with their clients. They can join together in despairing over the state of the male-dominated world. This may bring about a sense of solidarity that is helpful, but only for a while. It ceases to be helpful if the despair remains, rather than moving into something more creative. There is a real difficulty when neither helper or client can see any possibility of hope.

The development of feminist counselling and therapy

Feminist counselling is not a technique. It cannot be learnt in a workshop. It reflects, rather, a way of being, believing and understanding. In this way it is a perspective, not a technique, that arises from many sources that flow into, and feed, one another. It is essentially a perspective that allows fluidity, acknowledges interconnectedness, and encourages exploration. Feminist counselling attempts to avoid dogma, rigidity and jargon. It is concerned with making the counselling process accessible and comprehensible, rather than mystifying and mysterious. There is a commitment to an egalitarian relationship, rather than one that is embedded firmly in a hierarchical mode. Often there is an assumption that the counsellor–client relationship is inevitably, and necessarily, hierarchical. Jocelyn Chaplin challenges the belief in this inevitability:

Too often equality gets confused with sameness. The client and the counsellor are not the same; they have separate and different roles. But the counsellor is not there to dominate or have power over the client.... Feminist counselling aims instead to empower people and help them develop more self-confidence and control over their own lives. The counsellor is not seen as the expert or the doctor; the client is not a patient. Rather, they are two different people using clues to explore the life of one of them.[17]

Perhaps those who insist on the inevitability of a hierarchical relationship do so because they need to maintain their own power. Moving away from hierarchies can be deeply threatening, especially to those whose sense of self is dependent on a clearly defined role within such a structure. For such, the feminist approach, stemming from an entirely different philosophy, remains anathema.

Feminist counselling attracts and incorporates practitioners from a variety of theoretical backgrounds—psychodynamic, behavioural or humanistic. They may use art therapy and psychodrama. The use of symbols to allow exploration of the self is increasingly widespread. Similarly, feminist counsellors and therapists will represent a range of political beliefs and ideologies. They share common ground, but they are also able to tolerate differences. The development of a feminist perspective leads to some shared conclusions, but a variety of paths lead there. The common ground consists of a basic belief in the creation of an egalitarian relationship. Shared responsibility is encouraged. Another essential and central common thread is to incorporate the political stance into the therapeutic. This arises from a belief in the need for political and structural changes, and the recognition that societal realities are a major cause of women's unhappiness. There is a rejection of the 'adjustment' model which encourages women to adjust to society's demands. The inclusion of the political is a difference between feminist therapies, and those that attempt to be non-sexist:

Although feminist and non-sexist therapies are often used interchangeably, we make a distinction between the two. The major distinction is that feminist therapy incorporates the political values and philosophy of feminism... while non-sexist therapy does not... Non-sexist therapists may function in an egalitarian model also, but they do so from humanistic motivations and not, as feminist therapists, from a political position.[18]

Although the feminist approach incorporates a political perspective, this does not preclude clients from taking responsibility for aspects of their lives over which they do have some control. In order for women to be empowered and enabled to take greater charge of their own lives, they need to be able to differentiate the personal from the structural. It is important that women are able to identify aspects of their world over which they have control, and, equally, understand those that arise from being in an essentially sexist society. This opens the door to controlling and changing some parts of their lives. But other parts may not be amenable to change. Knowing which is which, placing responsibility firmly where it belongs, taking charge of what is theirs, and saying 'no' to what is not, is a huge step forward for women.

Encouraging women to trust themselves, to become more assertive, and to be able to acknowledge and express anger are other central themes in feminist work. Women's experience is heard; it is not invalidated or repressed. It is seen as an essential part of their being. It is recognized that their experience comes from an interaction of the internal and the external, but the first step in untangling this is allowing and encouraging the expression of that experience. Understanding cannot take place without providing an atmosphere conducive to trust, the freedom to say anything, and the belief that what is said will be accepted. This is not to say that feminist counselling is not challenging. It is. But the challenge to the client takes place within a context where her own view of her own world is not dismissed. By enabling her own perceptions to see the light of day, often for the first time, she can be helped to begin to redefine herself and her world. She may begin to develop a sense of her self less dependent on, and more separate from, her relationships with others. She may become more able to care for and nurture herself, as well as the others she has been brought up to care for.

Feminism in counselling and therapy has brought about a far greater awareness of the impact of gender in the therapeutic process. That, in itself, is an immensely valuable contribution, and one that has been sadly lacking in the traditional treatment of women. But it does far more than that. It issues a challenge to the existing organization of society. In that way it is often not a comfortable position to adopt; it does not fit in with existing structures, and is thereby resisted by those who are comfortable within them. For the many women who work within the confines of male-dominated institutions, it can feel frustrating and isolated. However, it is also exciting and hopeful, and marks a radical movement away from psychological and mental health provision that has quite astonishing difficulty in understanding issues basic to women, to their own organizations, and to society.

Male counsellors and female clients

Are we saying, then, that women clients should only be seen by women? While some would say a definite 'yes' to this, others may be less certain. Given the treatment that has been offered to women, it is understandable that services run by women for women are the choice for many. It seems absolutely essential that women should always have that option available. However, the reality is that for many the choice is not available. In some parts of the country women who cannot afford private counselling or therapy simply have to take what is available, and inevitably that means that some will be seen by a man. So what will that experience be like for the woman client? What might be the advantages? What might be the disadvantages? How do women themselves feel about the possibility of therapy or counselling with a man?

When the different possible gender combinations in counselling was discussed with a group of women, there was a unanimous feeling that a male counsellor and female client was the most risky and dangerous pairing. It was felt that it could be a relationship that had potential for extreme destructiveness, although it was also felt that the opposite could be true – that if it worked well it could be very constructive. There was a concern that physical attractiveness could be a problem, and might be acted out. Interestingly, this was not felt to be a difficulty in a pairing of a female therapist and male client – the risk of acting out was seen as minimal. It was felt that a female counsellor was more likely to contain such feelings, and less likely to act on them. These different perceptions of opposite-sex pairings are worth further comment. It was thought that while a male client was likely to have had previous experience of a woman who listened and took notice, a woman client may well experience her therapist as the first man to take her seriously. Small wonder, then, if she fell in love with him. The expectation that a woman counsellor or therapist would not give way to sexual feelings about a male client is also interesting. It seems to reflect another stereotype: that men are unable to contain their sexual urges, whereas women must and do.

Concern was also expressed that a chauvinistic attitude could come into play – that the man might have limited expectations of women, and that this would somehow be communicated in the relationship, to the detriment of the woman. There was also a fear that stereotypical attitudes would underline the process, and that one effect of this would be not to allow expression of anger. Some women felt that discussion of very intimate aspects of their lives might be difficult with a man. It was felt that stereotypes could interfere the other way around – that a woman could expect the male counsellor to rescue her (the 'knight in shining armour' myth) – that is, the man would be protective and not challenge. Both counsellor and client could collude in this type of process. It was recognized that a man working as a therapist should be sufficiently in touch with these issues to be able to work with them, rather than to collude.

On the more positive side, it was felt that a male therapist could provide a good role model of a man who would not exploit or abuse; that he could demonstrate an awareness and interest in women's issues; and that he would be able to acknowledge and challenge sexism both in himself and at a societal and structural level. It was felt, for instance, that it could be very healing, for a woman with a history of abuse by a man, to experience a relationship in which she could safely express her distress and anger, and find it both safe to do so and taken seriously. Women who have had a good therapeutic relationship with a male therapist, speak of it as a very rich, valuable and important experience. The experiences of this group of women must be heard, too, and be taken seriously. However, that recognition does not obliterate the real anxieties, expressed by many women, about the potential risks of seeing a male counsellor. Men need to be aware of these concerns. They need to consider them carefully and seriously in the light of their own practice. It is not sufficient for men simply to place themselves in the 'I'm a good guy' category. Such complacency is too easy, and often is not totally honest. Male counsellors need to scrutinize their own attitudes carefully in an ongoing way. Many women fear that they fail to do this, and that they will suffer the consequences.

So far, we have examined what women think about male counsellors. How does this match up with studies examining this same question? The answer is 'very closely indeed'. Studies have

shown that sexual relationships between male therapist and
female client are relatively common.[19] It is also unanimously
agreed that such relationships are harmful to the woman, and,
presumably, as male therapists have also read the literature, there
will be some who do not disclose their activities. So it could be
assumed that this is more frequent than the studies suggest. It is
also known that sex occurs between female therapist and male
client, but to a much lesser degree.[20] Neither is it uncommon for
therapists to marry their clients. How successful those marriages
are is unclear. It does seem, however, essentially different to be
committed to a long-term relationship than to a short-term one
based on seduction and exploitation. It also appears that for
women in that situation the sexual fantasy is better than the
reality. Virginia Davidson comments that: 'Seductive male therapists have unenviable track records as lovers, suffering frequently
from impotence and premature ejaculation.'[21]

Anna Seiden examines the evidence from research, and questions its implications for clinical practice. She points out that
misuse of the therapeutic relationship has a devastating effect on
women. In addition, she states that there is evidence that therapy
simply recreates the experience of so many women in their
marriages; that is, that they are in a 'one down' position, with the
male therapist having the monopoly of power, influence and
knowledge. In this way therapy is 'encouraging the fantasy that an
idealised relationship with a more powerful other is a better
solution to life problems than taking autonomous actions'.[22]

Research seems to back up the feelings of women – further
evidence, if it is needed, that when women are listened to they
have some accurate perceptions. Women need to be encouraged to
listen to themselves, and to find, if they are fortunate enough to
have a choice, the therapist or counsellor that they feel comfortable with. For some, this will be a man; others will prefer a woman.
If a male therapist is seen, it is obvious that he must have the high
degree of integrity that one could reasonably hope for and expect.

Women counsellors and women clients

When we ask how women perceive this combination, it is
immediately obvious that it is seen very differently from that of a
male counsellor and female client. The overall feeling is that
whatever else happens, at the end of the process the client would
be safe and not damaged. It is felt that it would be much easier to

talk about everything, and that there would be no forbidden or forbidding areas. A woman counsellor is likely to be more tuned into issues to do with children (even if she does not have any herself), to conflicting demands and expectations, and to questions relating to sexuality. There is a sense that time would not be wasted with a woman; that there would be a sufficient degree of shared experience to ensure more immediate understanding. Some women feel that there are some aspects of being a woman that are simply invisible to a man, and that cannot be made visible. It is just not part of a masculine way of seeing. The possibility of looking at mother–daughter relationships is also seen as an advantage of this pairing. Overall, it is felt that the relationship between female counsellor and female client can be very good and beneficial, with less hurdles to overcome.

However, it is felt that there can be difficulties. There is a danger of the relationship becoming too cosy and potentially collusive. It is recognized that there is a danger of falling into stereotypical patterns as much as in the male–female combination. Women do not always and automatically get on with one another. They, too, can be competitive, while feeling that they should not. Issues of power do arise; the female client can perceive the female counsellor as someone in a position of power and authority. It might be hard to express anger towards a woman. Earlier messages may reinforce this: 'don't shout at your mother', 'don't upset your mother', and 'little girls don't fight'. The client may fear that to be angry with a woman counsellor could either damage the counsellor, or result in the withdrawal of love. Of course, the other side of this anxiety is that a female counsellor provides an opportunity to understand, work through, and resolve these feelings, showing that anger and conflict can be part of one person, and of a relationship, without harming either.

Rebecca Goz echoes a widely held belief when she says:

> The request for a woman therapist by a woman patient is, in some major form or other, nearly always a disguised request by the patient to duplicate, review, reinstate, re-enact, repair and recreate some powerful unresolved tensions in relationship to her mother.[23]

The bringing up of girls primarily by their mothers produces complex difficulties for the former, in terms of separateness and independence.[24] In therapy, this central and crucial issue gives rise to a whole set of dynamics in client–therapist interactions. Given the centrality of the mother–daughter relationship to the woman's self-development, this aspect of a female pairing is of particular importance. Both partners in the all-female therapeutic relationship tend to see this as somehow a natural and inevitable issue that women will bring to counselling and therapy, and one that is less likely, and somehow more inappropriate, to be worked with in a different-gender pairing.

Experience indicates that many women prefer to see a woman, and this seems equally true in medicine and counselling. As we have seen, there is a concern that men may misuse their power, and that they cannot really grasp the experience of being a woman. In my earlier discussion of feminist therapy, I stressed that it is essential to this approach to understand the connections between the personal and the political. But not all female counsellors are feminist. This raises the question: are women in general more aware of both stereotyping and issues that effect women? The answer seems to be that they are. Even when women do not actively incorporate a political perspective into their work, their experiences of living in society tend to inform their practice, and give them another layer of awareness, less easily available to men. Judith Worrell takes up this point: 'Female counsellors have also been shown to be more aware of sex-stereotyped practices than male counsellors and are frequently more liberated than males in their attitudes towards expanded roles for women.'[25]

It can be very valuable to be part of a relationship in which two women are working together towards understanding and resolving a difficulty, without needing the assistance of a man. This is particularly evident in organizations such as women's therapy centres which are entirely run by women. The impact on a woman of being in such a centre should not be underestimated. Not only are they welcoming places – important in itself – but the ethos of a women-only organization is immediately communicated. For many, this will be their first experience of women being responsible for, and capable of, the overall running of a service.

The overriding comment that has to be made is that the care of women in British mental health services leaves much to be desired. Elizabeth Howell sums this up as follows:

> It is hard to fathom how the mental health establishment (which treats mainly women) could so underestimate the importance of issues that are relevant to the treatment of women, such as the characteristically patriarchal structure of the treatment situation.[26]

Counselling and therapy have a better track record: there is more awareness of women's issues, although individual practitioners need to examine their own sexism and stereotyping. There is a dire need for a very basic shift of attitude to be incorporated into all service provision. Men, and a male-dominated psychology, should not be seen as a prototype for the whole human race. Male assumptions should not dominate services mainly used by women. Women should be seen, heard, and listened to. They are not merely a supporting cast; they are central figures, and must be allowed to move out of the shadows.

Notes

1 Stricker, J. (1977). 'Implications of research for psychotherapeutic treatment of women', *American Psychologist*, 32.
2 Tennov, D. (1976). *Psychotherapy: The Hazardous Cure.* New York: Anchor Press/Doubleday, p. 191.
3 Melville, J. (1984). *The Tranquilliser Trap.* Fontana.
4 Gayford, J. (1978). 'Battered Wives' in Martin, J.P. (ed.) *Violence in the Family.* John Wiley.
5 Showalter, E. (1987). *The Female Malady: Women, Madness, and English Culture 1830–1980.* Virago, p. 249.
6 Broverman, I., Broverman, D., Clarkson, F., Rosenkrantz, P. and Vogel, S. (1970). 'Sex role stereotypes and clinical judgements of mental health', *Journal of Consulting Psychology*, 34. Reprinted in Howell, E. and Bayes, M. (eds), *Women and Mental Health.* New York: Basic Books, p. 92.
7 Laing, R.D. and Esterson, A. (1964). *Sanity, Madness, and the Family.* Tavistock Publications.
8 Cooper, C. (1971). *The Death of the Family.* Penguin.
9 Berke, J. (1979). *I Haven't Had to Go Mad Here.* Penguin; Berke, J. and Barnes, M. (1973). *Mary Barnes: Two Accounts of a Journey Through Madness.* Penguin.
10 Goffman, E. (1963). *Stigma.* Englewood Cliffs, N.J.: Prentice-Hall; Goffman, E. (1961). *Asylums.* Penguin.
11 Equal Opportunities Commission. (1987). *Women and Men in Britain: A Statistical Profile.* HMSO.
12 Dinnerstein, D. (1987). *The Rocking of the Cradle and the Ruling of the World.* The Women's Press.
13 Mitchell, J. (1971). *Women's Estate*, Penguin; Mitchell, J. (1975). *Psychoanalysis and Feminism.* Penguin.
14 Miller, J. Baker (1978). *Towards a New Psychology of Women.* Penguin.
15 Chodorow, N. (1978). *The Reproduction of Mothering.* University of California Press.
16 Eichenbaum, L. and Orbach, S. (1983). *What Do Women Want?* Michael Joseph; Eichenbaum, L. and Orbach, S. (1985). *Understanding Women.* Penguin.

17   Chaplin, J. (1988). *Feminist Counselling in Action.* Sage Publications, p. 7.
18   Rawlings, E. and Carter, D. (1977). 'Feminist and Non-sexist Psycho-therapy' in Rawlings, E. and Carter, D. (eds), *Psychotherapy for Women.* Springfield, Illinois: Charles C. Thomas.
19   Chesler, P. (1972). *Women and Madness.* New York: Doubleday; Dahlberg, C. (1970). 'Sexual contact between patient and therapist', *Contemporary Psychoanalysis*, 6, pp. 107–24; Masters, W.H. and Johnson, V.E. (1970). *Human Sexual Inadequacy.* Boston: Little Brown.
20   Perry, J.A. (1976). 'Physicians' erotic and non-erotic physical involvement with patients', *American Journal of Psychiatry.* 133, pp. 838–40.
21   Davidson, V. (1981). 'Psychiatry's Problem with No Name: Therapist–Patient Sex' in Howell, E. and Bayes, M. (eds.) *Women and Mental Health.* Basic Books: New York.
22   Seiden, A. (1976). 'Overview: Research on the psychology of women. Women in families, work, and psychotherapy', *American Journal of Psychiatry*, 133.
23   Goz, R. (1981). 'Women Patients and Women Therapists: Some Issues that come up in Psychotherapy', in Howell, E. and Bayes, M. (eds) *Women and Mental Health.* New York: Basic Books.
24   Orbach, S. and Eichenbaum, L. (1987). 'Separation and Intimacy' in Ernst, S. and Maguire, M. (eds), *Living with the Sphinx.* The Women's Press.
25   Worrell, J. (1981). 'New Directions in Counselling Women' in Howell, E. and Bayes, M. (eds), *Women and Mental Health.* New York: Basic Books.
26   Howell, E. (1981). 'Where Do We Go From Here?', in Howell, E. and Bayes, M. (eds), *Women and Mental Health.* New York: Basic Books.

5

Women's identity: pregnancy, mothering and motherhood

Before you are conceived
  I wanted you
Before you were born
  I loved you
Before you were here an hour
  I would die for you
This is the miracle of life.

Maureen Hawkins

The experience of carrying a new and growing life inside the body, and of giving birth, is a uniquely female experience. It gives credence to the concept of womb envy, and does little to encourage belief in penis envy. What could be more enviable than the ability to carry and bear a new being? The ability to have children is essential and central to how women define themselves. It is also central to ideologies and policies that relate to women which, in turn, greatly affect the course of their lives. Whether or not an individual woman decides to have children, the existence of this as a possibility is inevitably a significant question.

Those who are unable to have a child, or who do not wish to do so, can be left feeling that they swim against the tide of maternal instinct that somehow they should possess. Some reach this position from choice; others do not. They may feel a need to explain their situation; or that an unasked question is often left hanging in the air. Society assumes, first, that a woman will be in a relationship with a man, and second, that, being in one, she will then want a child. If she apparently does not, the response may be sympathy, surprise, or suspicion, openly expressed or otherwise. But there will be a question mark over her. For women who remain single, or who are in lesbian relationships, the situation is more complex. Approval of so-called maternal instinct and child-birth is closely linked to approved social situations. Long-stay wards of surviving older-style psychiatric hospitals still contain elderly women admitted in their youth having had an 'Illegitimate' child. The stigma of hospital admission, conveniently invisible to family and friends, was the lesser of the two unacceptable social evils. Thankfully, having a child outside marriage no longer evokes this response. However, the excitement that so often accompanies the announcement of pregnancy still tends to be muted if the mother is single or lesbian.

Daughters, because they are brought up by mothers, grow with the understanding that this role is part of the female identity. This is heavily reinforced by the world around them. The interpretation of how a 'good' mother should be is subject to changes relating to society's needs, rather than to considerations of good childcare practices. Women, therefore, grow up knowing that whatever else the future holds for them, and however important it becomes, it will be peripheral to the core of their being – defined as the ability to bear a child. Not fulfilling this criterion for acceptable womanhood, for whatever reason, creates an uneasiness for others even when the woman herself has resolved the issue. In the same way as single parenthood, and children born to an unmarried mother, do not carry the stigma of even one generation ago, the decision to remain childless or the inability to have a child may in time become more acceptable, and less questionable. In the 1990s it remains an issue both for women in that situation, and for the world around them. Issues relating to mothering arise in many different ways in counselling and therapy, and the following are a few examples. The complexities of trying to respond to the demands and needs of children, while at the same time meeting one's own, is a common difficulty, and one we will look at later in the chapter. It is particularly highlighted for single parents, though not exclusively so. Lesbian women, separated from male partners, live with the anxiety of losing custody of their children if this becomes disputed. This does occur, and the loss of care of their children often results in depression. Lesbian women who have not yet had children face a difficult decision. If they have children, they can fear both losing them and the possibility of the child becoming teased and ridiculed by an unsympathetic society. Women who cannot have children often experience grief and crises of identity. This can occur, for example when infertility is diagnosed, or during middle age with the recognition that it is too late to have a child. Such issues may represent the core of the difficulties a woman brings to counselling, or can be peripheral, though still significant. Understanding mothering as central to women's identity is crucial when issues such as these are in evidence, as they frequently are.

The effects of pregnancy, childbirth and child upbringing

Relationship with the self

If not having a child is problematic, what can be said of the experience of having a child? Unlike other experiences, and other relationships – which may, or may not, endure – it lasts a lifetime. Becoming pregnant brings about changes; some immediate, others delayed; some expected and enjoyed, others unpleasant, frightening, or simply surprising. These changes encompass all aspects of the woman's self and her world, and continue from that point on, as the child is born and develops through babyhood, to childhood and into adulthood.

In pregnancy the woman's relationship with herself undergoes rapid change. Even if she is delighted to be pregnant, and eagerly awaiting the birth, the process is something of a shock. No longer is she alone with her body; she finds herself sharing it with a new and growing person. Pregnancy is a strangely intimate relationship with another. It is the ultimate in symbiosis. Unless a decision is taken not to continue with the pregnancy, or miscarriage occurs, the baby will continue to grow, and the expected date of delivery moves inexorably closer. Advancing pregnancy makes the reality of the baby more and more visible to everyone. As her body continues to change and grow in tune with her child, so do the boundaries of her self change, both literally, in a physical sense, and in a deeply psychological sense. With the birth comes the awareness that this new person has an identity, personality and temperament all of his/her own, while still, somehow, being connected and attached to the mother.

Prior to birth, the act of sharing one body may have been comfortable, exciting, wondrous and enjoyable. It may have been uncomfortable, unpleasant, invasive and hard to tolerate. Most women seem to experience aspects of both. While some really do appear to float through pregnancy in the state of glorious and beautiful rapture depicted in so many advertisements, others drag themselves around feeling ill, irritable and exhausted. For the latter group, childbirth itself can feel a welcome relief from the awfulness of pregnancy. But it may not: giving birth can be felt as an enormous loss by some women.

Birth, if all goes well, is often a joyous occasion, but it can awaken or reinforce confusion over self-identity. A difficulty that is expressed frequently by women in counselling and therapy is encapsulated in the experience of childbirth. There is a deep and perplexing confusion: how is it possible to be both separate and to maintain intimacy and connectedness? Are the two essentially incompatible, with the loss of one aspect needed in order satisfactorily to sustain the other? Childbirth often turns the spotlight on this dilemma. For a few women, the confusion becomes chaos, and very severe depression and disturbance results. Others experience less serious difficulties, but therapists and counsellors need to be aware that women are particularly psychologically vulnerable at this time.

Pregnancy and medical care

Having a baby is often the first time that previously healthy women experience prolonged contact with the medical profession. Those who are cared for by their own family doctor will have a far greater degree of consistency of care, and the opportunity to get to know the person caring for them. Many women do not have this service available to them and become accustomed to long waits in hospital ante-natal clinics. Studies[1] have shown how difficult it is for expectant mothers either to ask questions they wish to ask or to have the opportunity to become safely familiar with those who will attend the birth. At a time when women are likely to experience anxiety, and need access to accurate information, this is very unsatisfactory. Additionally, given potential or actual confusion over identity at this time, hospital care erodes this even further. Long waits, lack of information, scant privacy and crowded waiting rooms can turn excitement and anticipation into an endurance test. When the expectant mother should be feeling special, she becomes another product on the conveyor belt, and her identity slips even further away.

In some ways it is because ante-natal care is so task-centred that a person becomes lost. A first-time expectant mother described how she was left in a cubicle, told to undress, given a gown that she had to clutch around her to keep it closed, and left there. She then heard the consultant leave the next cubicle; discuss another patient in her hearing, before going off for a cup of tea. Half an hour later he returned and she was examined. She felt angry, deserted and entirely insignificant. There was no apology, and no explanation for the delay. As Barbie Antonis points out:

A contradiction exists between the notion that bearing a child is the highest goal a woman can achieve and the low marginal status in which she finds herself when pregnant and a mother.[2]

Nurses and doctors who work in these medical settings would do well to remember that the application of some very basic counselling skills could be valuably employed. Listening carefully to what is being said, and responding in an appropriate manner, need take no more time, yet the quality of patient care will be considerably enhanced. Similarly, respecting confidentiality, and always ensuring its maintenance, are crucial to the patient's confidence in those caring for her. It should also be remembered that for women who are not part of a traditional couple relationship, the stresses and feelings of alienation may be even greater. It is clear that even middle-class women, used to dealing with professionals, and often professionals themselves, find difficulty in being heard in this situation. How much more problematic it is then, for women not used to asserting themselves, or for those from a minority cultural background.

Relationships with others

For the woman, the relationship that will most obviously change in focus, during and after pregnancy, is the one with her partner. This is particularly so with a first child. To adjust from living as two adults, with the freedom that entails, to sharing your life and home with a small and demanding person, is a major change for both. For the woman it is frequently accompanied by a change of economic status which, perhaps for the first time, makes her financially dependent on her partner. Issues of dependency and independency are therefore likely to arise. If she returns to work shortly after the birth (and it should be remembered that most mothers of very small children do not work in full-time paid employment), her status will have changed. Even if she is in full-time work, she will most likely carry the practical and emotional responsibility for care of the baby, and she will often feel she is struggling to meet all these demands adequately. She may accept this as part of her role, or she may experience resentment towards her less involved partner. She may vacillate between these responses, but inevitably the relationship with him will undergo change. Practically, she will have less time and be more tired. Emotionally, a considerable amount of her resources will be given to her baby, and it may be difficult for her to achieve a balance between that and her relationship with her partner.

The delight women can experience with their very young children does not preclude their awareness that having a child turns their world upside-down and inside-out. Male partners share in the impact of this experience. However, the intensity and amount of change in lifestyle and experience of self it induces is not comparable. Women feel that childbirth changes them in essential ways, and this, combined with their involvement in the new relationship with the baby, can cause disruption and difficulty in their partnership or marriage. Just as children leaving home causes couples to reassess their relationship, so does the arrival of children, and both situations can bring individuals or couples to counselling.

Other relationships similarly undergo change. Friendships with women who are childless, and who, as a result, have a freer lifestyle, are affected. There will be less experience in common, and a small child places restraints on both ease of mobility and finances. Mothers tend to be drawn into a world of other mothers. This may be experienced as deeply pleasurable and truly supportive, or as somewhat restrictive, or even as both. But it is certainly a different world, with a different basis, and can again focus the woman on thoughts of who she actually is.

The new mother's relationships with female members of both her and her partner's family, and particularly with her own mother, are also likely to alter. For some women it is like finally being allowed into an exclusive club: they have now met the criteria for membership. There is a shared language and experience, which can be both comforting and conflictual. Advice is not always wanted or agreed with, but, for instance, the discovery that others really understand the meaning of true exhaustion can be a great relief. Unresolved difficulties with her own mother may resurface in an unexpectedly sharp and painful way at this stage of a new mother's life. As her child grows older, difficult experiences from the mother's own childhood can be awakened or reawakened into unpleasant activity. Again, these experiences and feelings are frequently presented by women seeking counselling help.

Motherhood and paid employment

Mothers who go out to work face conflicting demands on their time and resources. This conflict between the demands of work and the needs of children is central to the lives of many women. Women may work for personal satisfaction, whilst many do so from financial necessity. Whatever the motive, women frequently end up with a double workload. The two accounts that follow, from women in very different social situations, illustrate their long working day. For these two the balance is maintained. They are not unhappy or dissatisfied; they have in common a sense of fulfilment, but the issues involved in this way of life are evident in both accounts. Both reinforce the theme (that will be explored in the following chapter) of paid work being protective to women, while simultaneously demanding huge resources of energy and organization.

Sarah, a translator, works from home, and has two daughters. The older is aged three years, and the baby is three months. She describes her day:

> My day? Well, I get up at six. I feed the baby, and I do the washing. Hopefully she'll go back to sleep for a while. Then the other one wakes up, and I'll dress her, and we'll have breakfast. My husband goes off to work. If it's my turn I'll take Paula to play group along with three others. If it's not my turn she'll be collected. Then I'll bath the baby, and with any luck she'll go in her pram for a while and I'll do some work. Luckily she's a very peaceful baby. At twelve o'clock Paula comes back and the next few hours are taken up with meals, shopping, going to the park, visiting friends and playing. And more meals. At six my husband comes home, and he'll play with Paula and bath her whilst I cook our meal. I try and get the baby to bed, often not very successfully. And then I really have to get down to work. If the baby hasn't settled then I'll have her on one arm whilst I write or type. If my husband isn't working he'll take her for a while, but he can only do one or the other, I've got used to doing both at once. She'll usually settle by about ten, and I'll work undisturbed until about twelve. She still often wakes a couple of times in the night and it's me who sees to her. My husband is always dead to the world, and if I wake him and insist he goes, by that time she'll be screaming blue murder, so there's not much point. It is hard work, but I enjoy my job and the children, and at least I work from home and don't feel anxious about them.

The following account is from a young woman, a single parent with boys of two and three. She is a semi-skilled factory worker.

> I have to get up really early. Luckily the nursery is near here. It's better now they've got places. I can push them there in the pushchair. But I hate having to wake them, it seems all wrong, they look so sleepy and peaceful, and in the winter it's so cold. But I do know they're well looked after, and safe and happy. It's awful if they're ill. It really hurts leaving them then. Oh, but it's better than

being on the social. It is hard work though. A man wouldn't know, would he? I try and do the shopping in my lunch hour, and the washing and cleaning get done somehow. And when I fetch them back they want me to play. I want to, and I'm real pleased to see them, but I'd love just to sit down. It can pull you to pieces if you let it. But I do manage, and that's a really good feeling. When I was with their dad he didn't do anything anyway, and he used to scare us. So it's really easier, but it's a bit lonely.

Listening to women describe their working day is frequently impressive, although they themselves see nothing unusual about it. In many ways that reflects the reality: there is nothing unusual, because this is how women with children live. Organization and timing are crucial, as is the ability to flexibly switch from one task to another, or to do several simultaneously. It is a very different way of life to living either alone or with a partner. It is an adjustment that carries with it many issues related to a woman's individual psychology; to her relationship with her partner if she has one (or, if she has not, with others related to her single parenthood); and to her relationship with the wider world. These adjustments start with pregnancy and childbirth, but children are an ongoing process, not a one-off event, and as they grow older different responses and adjustments become necessary.

Motherhood and the growing child

We saw in Chapter 1 the significance for Suzanne of her children growing older. When children reach a certain age their mothers are often reminded of their own experiences of life at that age. This can bring back pleasant memories, but it may do the opposite. For instance, a woman with a ten-year-old daughter presented herself for counselling. She described panic and anxiety attacks that revolved around an extreme fear that she would not be able to continue caring for her child. She also described how, if she felt she was not a good mother, she would be nothing, that she would dissolve. A previous counsellor had felt that she needed psychiatric treatment, and this had increased her fear. Indeed, her symptoms were so considerable, and her description of them so graphic, that in another setting a psychotic or 'borderline personality' label may well have become attached. She felt that her own sense of her reality and her self was sliding away.

After some time working with her, it transpired that when she herself was ten, her own mother had been very ill, and had been rushed into hospital and received lengthy treatment. She made a good recovery after a long period of convalescence, but during this time the whole family, including her young daughter, had to take special care of her. In many ways the roles had been reversed, the daughter becoming the mother. One aspect of this experience that had been repressed until this time was that during her mother's stay in hospital, she was cared for by family friends. She had been very frightened by the father in the household, who made sexual suggestions and remarks to her that she could not fully understand but felt 'sickened' by. She could not tell anyone, and described feelings at the time of 'losing herself', of 'disappearing' and 'not existing'. It became clear that at the age of ten she experienced two very disturbing events. She felt that her world, as she knew it, had disappeared, that her childhood had ended precipitously, and she took refuge inside herself. This self, in many ways, became paralysed. It did not 'dissolve' or 'disappear', but it certainly was forced into hibernation. There are many relevant levels to this woman's story. Had she gone for psychiatric help, there is the obvious question of whether hospital admission would have taken place. A large chunk of history would then have been repeated, for both mother and daughter, possibly without acknowledgement or the opportunity to work through it.

As it happened, this was avoided: had it not been, another damaging experience might have reinforced earlier fears. Again, the woman could have been in a situation over which she had no control of her destiny. Her experiences at this time in many ways recreated her own ten-year-old world, which had been successfully put away from conscious memory. The needy child in her emerged, carrying with it a complexity of unexpressed feelings of desertion, incomprehension, guilt, terror, rage and grief. These had to be dealt with within the context of continuing to care for her own growing daughter, who had needs of her own and was frightened by her mother's obvious distress. Her mother, terrified that her daughter would suffer similarly, and feeling that if this happened her reason for being would disappear, found her panic intensifying. The more panic she experienced, the less in control she felt, and a vicious downward spiral rapidly emerged.

Until she was able to start making sense of her current feelings in terms of her past experiences, she was effectively paralysed by them. Enabling understanding and safe expression of her feelings was the start of movement out of paralysis into autonomous activity. It is also interesting to note that neither her own father nor her daughter's father were able to be actively involved in supporting their children at a difficult time. If she had been hospitalized, her child would have needed to be cared for by someone else; her husband, like her father before him, had a job that entailed travelling away from home.

This story illustrates how the mother–child bond can provoke or uncover powerful feelings for women. Of course, many do not have such disturbing memories of their own childhood, although they can often be surprised by the flashbacks that children can evoke. What is common to all mothers is that, having made initial alterations to lifestyle and self with the birth of a child, many more have to be made as the child grows older and enters different stages of development. The initial separation at birth is followed by others. Stopping breastfeeding, the child's first foray into the world without mother, the start of school, the onset of adolescence, and finally leaving home, are all major stages which have to be traversed. As we have noted previously, mothering in Western society becomes firmly equated with motherhood. Whilst the latter is biologically determined, mothering is not. Until this changes, women will bear the brunt of the emotional impact of accompanying their children through these stages, emphasizing further for them the perplexing question of their own separateness, and their own connectedness.

So far, we have looked at the impact and meaning of pregnancy, birth and motherhood, with the assumption that this is a process that has progressed satisfactorily. This is not always the case, and for women who experience miscarriage, abortion, or stillbirth, the experience is vastly different.

Miscarriage and stillbirth

> After the third miscarriage I felt I was going mad. I thought, I'm not a proper woman, and, that I must have done something really bad to deserve this. Every month I'd wonder, am I pregnant. It dominated my life. I felt entirely alone; no one understood the agonies I was going through. When I finally got through a pregnancy and had my baby I was depressed. It was awful, everyone expected me to be ecstatic and there I was weeping all over everyone. She was a difficult baby and one day I found myself thinking, I don't like you. And I felt so guilty. The whole thing has just left me very unhappy and very guilty.

In many ways miscarriage is a hidden and often unrecognized loss for women. If often occurs when the fact of pregnancy is known only to the potential parents. A reality exists for them that is not acknowledged or seen by others. However, for the woman concerned the experience has been real; she has begun to carry a child, and has to cope with the grief of losing it. If it occurs later in pregnancy, it may be easier to share this with others and to receive some support, but the miscarriage itself is likely to be painful and unpleasant. For women who have been through this several times (and many have), anxiety, depression, and feelings of lack of self-worth are common. As illustrated above, women may feel that their female identity and value is threatened, and that somehow they must be bad. It can seem the only explanation for such a bad thing happening to them, an explanation which makes sense in the context of a world in which the ability to have a child is seen as both normal and desirable.

Women who do not enjoy a normal pregnancy are something of an anomaly for medical services, who do not seem to know quite what to do with them:

> A woman whose pregnancy does not result in the usual happy event presents embarrassing problems. There is no live baby to join the other squalling babies in the nursery, and the woman no longer qualifies as a mother – even if she has other children at home. She and her baby are misfits. The solution to this dilemma lies in disposing of the evidence as quickly as possible. After a 'rugger pass' to get rid of the baby, the mother has to be disposed of too. Usually she is put in a room by herself and sent home as fast as possible.[3]

A mother who has a stillborn child experiences a loss and trauma made worse by having carried her baby for longer. She will have made plans for the child, and purchased equipment. It will have become the focus of her life, of her partner's and close friends and family will also have been involved. She may have already left her job, or have been planning to. Many of the adjustments to pregnancy that we have noted have already been made; the birth will have taken place in a medical setting generally geared to happy events and the celebration of life, rather than grieving for death. A stillborn child is an enormous loss to both parents, but the mother has an existing relationship which cannot be directly or totally shared or experienced by the father. He has lost a new person that he was looking forward to knowing. The mother has lost someone who has already been an intimate part of her. Hers is a lonely grief. This loneliness is a particular aspect of the experience of any woman who has lost a child, for whatever reason, before it has enjoyed a separate existence. It is hard to say goodbye to someone you did not know, but loved dearly; who was still a stranger, while having the closest possible relationship with you. It is made harder by a world that decrees that your feminity is linked with successful childbearing.

Abortion

> This is the month, as I write, of warm flowery days and frosty nights when she would have been three. Sometimes in the dark with M inside me I can feel the place where she was and it makes me cry. Whether the tears are for grief or something quite different, I can't say.[4]

Abortion is not an easy option for women. It causes pain and agony that can reverberate for years, as the quotation above vividly captures. It is a decision taken for a variety of rationally correct reasons, and yet rarely feels right. Reasoning and rational thought do not coincide with feeling where abortion is concerned. This is illustrated by the words of a young woman of twenty who was convinced of the necessity of an abortion:

> I would fight for the right of a woman to decide whether or not she has a child. I don't believe that rubbish about murder. Those who argue that should take a good look at the world, and see just how much real murder goes on. But now I've had an abortion it doesn't feel like that. I haven't changed what I think at all. But I just keep wanting my baby back. I feel different. I feel empty and guilty, as though something has died. I don't know if that's because my baby is dead, or that a bit of me has died with it. It wasn't a wrong decision, I know that. But it's so sad.

Women who have experienced miscarriage or stillbirth know the agonies caused by self-recrimination. They ask themselves what they did to make this happen. After abortion, a similar feeling can be present, except that women in that situation are faced with the clear knowledge that it was their action that caused the pregnancy to cease. As with miscarriage, it is a lonely experience, even for women who have the support of a partner:

> We talked it over a lot and shed a lot of tears together and he couldn't have been more caring, more involved but even so I felt quite alone. It was my body, I had to have the abortion; I had to be the one to actually arrange it all.[5]

Some women are very alone at this time:

> I really wanted the baby but my boyfriend didn't and when I tried to persuade him he became very angry and so I knew there really wasn't any choice because I couldn't have managed alone. Once I had arranged the abortion I was so sad and unhappy and I had no one to tell as John said I couldn't tell anyone, no one must know. I only had myself and the thoughts were flowing through my mind and I couldn't sort them out at all.

Others find that a supportive partner at the time has a very short tolerance span after the abortion:

> Oh yes, he was all sympathy at the time, but he didn't understand that sort of thing just doesn't go away just to suit him. I think he saw it as a minor operation, and if there weren't any complications then there was no problem. It really hit me a year after, and he said he couldn't cope with me going on about it. I thought, lucky him, he has a choice. He can tell me to shut up and I have to. It's as though it's nothing to do with him; either the event or how I'm left feeling. It's an irritation to him; to me it was a loss of something precious. I know I couldn't have kept him and the baby. I think I might have chosen the wrong one.

A popular myth is that abortion is available on demand. It is not. It is legal, and the law is open to liberal interpretation, which may or may not happen. Some doctors make little secret of their disapproval of abortion, and of women who seek it. Others are supportive, genuinely caring, and helpful. It remains a question largely of luck whether a woman receives a helpful or a judgementally antagonistic response to her request. Women are 'free' to have abortions, but the power is left firmly in the hands of the medical hierarchy. This has led to huge anomalies, allowing individual doctors to decide according to their own individual bias, be it in relation to religion, race, class, physical appearance or marital status.[6]

It is clear that society has a considerable investment in women having children, and being responsible for their upbringing. This reassures and reinforces the whole basis of a patriarchal society, but how is this relevant to the process of counselling and therapy with women?

Motherhood: the implications for therapy and counselling

Understanding the context of women's lives

For whatever complex reasons, women are primarily defined as mothers and carers in a most tenacious way (see Chodorow[7] and Dinnerstein[8] for a detailed debate on this). Whether or not they become mothers, and most do, this definition affects their lives to a considerable extent. Those working with women need to be aware, first, of how this may manifest itself in the difficulties experienced by women, and second, of the impact of children on their lives.

Anxieties over dependency, in a society that makes it very difficult for women (particularly mothers) to be independent, are frequently expressed. Women may strive to become independent in an economic sense, yet few achieve this. They are left with the need to be cared for and nurtured, in a situation where this is also clearly their own role as well. In becoming a mother, and thereby entering the mothering role, a woman's own experience as a small child may surface. She may be able to identify this as the problem, but it can be expressed as feelings towards her own child, apparently unconnected with her own earlier experiences. This was seen earlier in the example of the woman with the ten-year-old daughter. In that instance, the counsellor recognized that the two may have been connected, and was able to ask her client if she felt able to talk about what her life had been like when she was that age. And slowly the story emerged. Without an awareness that patterns can repeat themselves in particular ways for women with children, it may not have been possible for such connections to be made.

Another central focus for many women is the difficulty in being themselves while also being a carer and mother. We have seen how this is reflected in a balancing act that often works, but sometimes does not. Counsellors need to be able to acknowledge the practical difficulties and the problems, as well as the demands imposed by society, while also being aware of underlying individual dynamics. Unravelling this is not easy, and the counsellor will not be able to facilitate this process without appreciating the total context in which it operates.

Understanding the different stages of a child's life, and the consequent ever-changing demands on a woman, is necessary if she is to believe her therapist is in the same world as her, and not on a different planet. Male counsellors need to be particularly careful about this. Women very readily invalidate their own experiences as mothers, and this can be rapidly reinforced if the counsellor is unaware, for example, of how it can feel when the youngest child starts school, or a pregnancy cannot be continued.

The ability of the counsellor to recognize the contradictions that relate to motherhood will assist the client's exploration of these contradictions. They are often uncomfortable to get close to, as they challenge the myths, particularly of glorious motherhood. Whatever the joys of mothering, and for many women these are quite unquantifiable but very real, this is only one part of reality. The rest of the picture cannot be ignored if women are to enter the whole world, rather than be tucked away in a corner.

Abortion counselling

Strong feelings abound regarding abortion. It is vital for any therapist or counsellor working in this field to have dealt with his/her own feelings on abortion and childbirth. This is an agonizing time for a woman, and she does not want to encounter a counsellor in the throes of his/her own moral angst. Counsellors should have come to terms with the personal issues involved. They need to believe in the right of a woman to make decisions for herself regarding her own body and her own child. Only then can the client be helped to look at how she feels, and to make her own decisions.

There is clearly a distinction to be made between pre-abortion and post-abortion counselling. The former is working in a crisis situation, in which limited time is available. A response has to be made quickly to the client, who in turn has to make a decision in a short space of time. Often in counselling, clients are encouraged towards taking time over major life decisions; pre-abortion counselling does not allow this. Emotional reactions need to be explored, and options examined. Time limits have to be noted and stated, without putting undue pressure on the client. It can be difficult simultaneously to affirm the reality of the need to decide, while also wanting to explore other avenues fully.

Women are sometimes wary of expressing their doubts, in case abortion is then denied, but the opportunity to express these and have them acknowledged is valuable. They need to be able to discuss ambivalent feelings, and may have to accept that a degree of ambivalence is inevitable and to be expected; few women can feel entirely at ease with the decision to abort. Given the relatively short time available, information needs to be readily available to the client. Again, many women are uneasy about asking, but they need to know the details of the procedure. It is important that counsellors are able to discuss these without tension or difficulty on their part. At this stage there is a focus on enabling the client to discover and use her own coping skills. It is a very difficult choice to make. For some women, it may be the first major decision they have ever taken alone, and they know they have to make it quickly.

Post-abortion counselling is free of time pressure, and there is no decision to make. Women can experience grief, anger, reactive depression and other feelings associated with loss. They may feel they have no right to feel any of these things, that it has been their fault; they took the decision, so they have no right to complain about the consequences. Women are very good at blaming themselves, and are especially adept at this when it comes to abortion. Women have a right to their feelings, and counselling can both enable expression of these and validate their right to have them. Abortion can produce enormous strain on the relationship that produced the pregnancy, and couple counselling may be helpful and appropriate. If a woman has had several abortions, this may need further exploration. It may be that unconscious factors are at work which, if not identified, may cause further and future repetitions.

Those who work in a medical setting – nurses, doctors, or social workers – may have no choice about being involved in abortion work, although they may have strong feelings of disapproval. Certainly, the experience of women undergoing abortion can be made more painful by judgemental and unsympathetic attitudes on the part of the staff. Women undergo considerable conflict when faced with unplanned and unwanted pregnancy. Greater awareness of this and sensitivity towards the dilemma could make the ordeal less harrowing. It should be remembered that women are vulnerable at this time; they can feel trapped in a situation where the right decision is also the wrong one. Abortion can seem like an invasion, and an attack on their bodies, and further attacks or assaults on them by uncaring staff are quite unjustified.

Miscarriage and stillbirth

Generally, considerable sympathy is felt towards women who suffer from miscarriage or stillbirth. They do not have to contend with the moral outrage that can be so vehemently expressed towards abortion. However, for many women sympathy is not enough, and, instead of being given time to grieve, their distress is repressed by platitudes. The advice to try to conceive another child soon may be well meant, but it invalidates the significance and importance of the child who has been lost.

Parents who have lost a child through miscarriage or stillbirth are bereaved, and like any other bereaved person need to be allowed to grieve. The mother will need support to re-establish her life on a different basis, at least for the time being. As with abortion, there is a need for accurate information, which may not have been given, or may not have been adequately and accurately heard at the time. It can be a valuable part of the counselling process in the early days, if the client is able to check out with the counsellor what is fact and reality, and what is fantasy and fear. This will not be an easy distinction to draw; fantasies are powerful and facts hard to assimilate.

The client may need to go over and over the experience time and time again, before she is able to begin leaving it behind her. As with any other grief, there will be anger, guilt, disbelief, depression and despair. None of this can be hurried, but support and acceptance of all these facets of grief will enable resolution finally to take place. If the woman is in a relationship, the relationship itself, and her partner, may be under considerable pressure. Consideration could be given to couple counselling, although in addition the woman may also need time alone with her counsellor. Those working in hospitals are in a position to offer an immediate response to what is an appalling crisis. This is, as we have seen, an extremely lonely time for a woman, and the availability of someone who will listen, and who will accept that it is a personal tragedy, can alleviate some of the aloneness. Particularly with a stillborn child, so recognizable as a baby, care and time must be taken to ascertain the parents' wishes. Holding the child, taking photos, saying hello and goodbye, and any other rituals that are requested must be provided. Parents should spend as long with the child as they wish, perhaps on several different occasions. Tidying the dead child away briskly and efficiently may enable staff to deal with the pain but it does not help the parents with their grief. Leaving hospital and going home is a particularly poignant time. It can be helpful if someone in a counselling role in the hospital is also able to visit at home. The need to talk through the experience can be helped if someone who was part of it is there.

A normal pregnancy and childbirth can be both enthralling and special, but also frightening and anxiety-provoking. It is a momentous event in the life of any woman. When all does not go well, it can feel as if the world is disintegrating. Although women are given powerful messages that motherhood is their *métier*, and are granted approval in this role, their treatment does not always encourage belief in these messages. Those working with women should recognize the enormity of the experience, and react accordingly. This does not stop at the birth of the child. If motherhood really is as precious and special as women are brought up to believe, this should be reflected in a far greater awareness of the psychological significance of this state. Therapists and counsellors, in their work with women, periodically need to ask themselves if they are sufficiently aware of the issues.

Notes

1 For example, see *Report on Ante-natal Care*, Cambridge Community Health Council, 1987.
2 Antonis, B. (1981). 'Mothering and Motherhood', in Cambridge Women's Studies Group (ed.), *Women in Society*. Virago, p. 63.
3 Lovell, A. 'When a baby dies', *New Society*, 4 August 1983, p. 167.
4 Hey, V. (ed.) (1989). *Hidden Loss*. The Women's Press, p. 14.
5 Neustatter, A. and Newson, G. (1986). *Mixed Feelings: The Experience of Abortion*. Pluto Press, p. 32.
6 Dana, M. (1987). 'Abortion—a woman's right to feel', in Ernst, S. and Maguire, M. (eds), *Living with the Sphinx*. The Women's Press, p. 155.
7 Chodorow, N. (1978). *The Reproduction of Mothering*. University of California Press.
8 Dinnerstein, D. (1987). *The Rocking of the Cradle and the Ruling of the World*. The Women's Press.

6

Women and depression

> I just want to sit and cry. I don't want to eat but sometimes I do
> because it fills the time. I don't want to sleep or I'll sleep all the
> time. I don't want to be alive, but it would take too much effort
> to plan to kill myself. Everything becomes completely out of
> control, it all goes too fast. It's like life is rushing on and
> dragging me kicking and screaming behind. It's like a dull
> empty ache inside; I can feel it physically. Then it can grow
> until it's an awful, awful pain and it takes over my whole self.
> It's like an enormous painful whole. And people say, 'Well, do
> something to distract yourself.' If you're in really awful pain it
> won't go away, you can't ignore it, because it becomes you – it *is*
> you. And it can get beyond pain, to a point where everything
> disappears, and I have disappeared and it's like I'm in space; in
> total darkness, unattached to anything, wandering in circles in
> the dark.

To anyone who has ever been depressed, this woman's description
of the pain and the hopelessness that is often experienced will be
familiar. Much is written on depression, and there is a great deal of
discussion as to its origins, its treatment and its meaning in
psychology, sociology, psychotherapy and medicine. Classifi-
cations and definitions are numerous: depression can be neurotic
or psychotic; reactive or endogenous; primary or secondary. The
sufferer may be seen as having a depressive personality, or may be
identified as having a smiling or hidden depression. A plethora of
such definitions can be discovered; a similar number of 'treat-
ments' can be identified. Depending on which of these happens to
be the medical or therapeutic flavour of the month, depressed
women can be on the receiving end of one of an enormous range of
techniques and interventions. How many of these actually take
into account the real nature of women's experience is highly
questionable.

However much depression may be ill defined and not fully
understood, it remains a painful reality that darkens the lives of
large numbers of women, and causes the sort of suffering, so
vividly described above, which is hard to convey to anyone who
has not experienced it personally. Although it is hard to describe as

a precise psychological condition, women, when invited to do so, are themselves able vividly to express the agonies and isolation caused by depression. Their widespread experience of depression is such that any discussion of women in counselling must give serious attention to this as an area of considerable concern.

Throughout the mental health field it is a fact that many more women than men present as depressed, and many more are diagnosed as such. This is true of out-patient clinics, in-patient admissions, community and other counselling services, and of women who visit their general practitioners. In all studies of depression women outnumber men by between two and six times.

It has been argued that women are more likely to seek help than men, and that this in itself inflates the figures. Indeed there is evidence that women do consult their doctors and use other medical and counselling services more than men. This cannot explain, however, the similarly high levels of depression that have been found in community studies of the general population. In their study of women in Camberwell, George Brown and Tirril Harris[1] found that 15 per cent of the women studied were depressed and another 18 per cent were identified as being on the borderline of depression. Close links were identified between depression and the quality (or rather, lack of it) of daily experience. There was only a very slight suggestion of the existence of a small subgroup of women in whom depression existed without an obvious causal factor. Their findings appear to contradict the various theories that support biological and chemical features in the genesis of depression. Instead, they suggest the need to look rather more closely at wider social and political processes.

Although all the studies tell us that at all ages the rates of depression are higher for women, there remain significant variations within this overall pattern. Rates of depression among all age groups of women are rising, but this is especially so among younger women. Particularly at risk are women who are at home with young children. This is of great concern; the quality of life for many young women is being adversely affected, and consequently the mental health of a generation of children is also being put at risk. Research by Naomi Richman,[2] studying a group of mothers of three-year-old children, showed that at least a third of these mothers had been significantly depressed in the year before her study. Similarly, Brown and Harris showed that a third of those mothers with pre-school children had been depressed at some time during the three months prior to their interview.

What else do such studies tell us? Brown and Harris also demonstrate that, subject to equivalent levels of stress, working-class women were five times more likely to be depressed than middle-class women. Four factors were found to be of particular importance. These were: loss of mother in childhood; three or more children living at home under the age of fourteen; the absence of a close and confiding relationship with a partner; and the lack of a full- or part-time job outside the home. The first three of these were more likely to be found among working-class women. It appears that class factors as well as gender issues are significant.

It is interesting to note that paid employment seems to be a protecting factor making women less vulnerable to depression. That this is so among mothers with young children is particularly important. Given the appalling lack of day care provision for the under-fives, of post-school and holiday care for over-fives in the UK, and the exhaustion so often experienced by mothers trying to cope with parenting and paid employment, this knowledge is illuminating. It is vividly illustrated through the words of a working mother interviewed by Sue Sharpe:

> I was a different person. I mean, I was on valium with terrible depressions previously and I was a different person altogether. I mean, I used to come out of that office feeling as if I'd achieved something, although I'd only have typed letters all afternoon. I felt as though I was part of the world again, because it was like solitary confinement, being at home all the time with the youngsters. It gave me a reason for living, just going to work, for getting up each day.[3]

If this is the situation for many younger women with children, how does this compare with women as they grow older? A typical stereotype of the depressed woman is someone who is meno-pausal and middle-aged, grieving for her lost youth and her lost children. Is this myth or reality? Certainly, for women of all ages hormonal changes can be a useful peg on which to hang the cause of depression, although this is an especially useful target for middle-aged women approaching the menopause. By listing menstruation (its onset and cessation), pre-menstrual tension, pre- and post-natal depression, as causes of depression in women, we provide a series of explanations that cover most years of a woman's life.

But this overemphasis on purely physical causation, is both

dangerous and convenient when used as a blanket explanation. It is dangerous because women are once more persuaded that they themselves and their bodies are somehow inferior and at fault. Men, created differently, are stronger, and somehow superior, because they do not appear to experience the same problems. The danger extends beyond this; as with any generalized and over-simplified explanation it can prevent a real and caring response to the whole person, even if some of her difficulties may, in part or in total, also have a hormonal basis.

It is, however, a convenient explanation. Society is not at fault; men do not carry any responsibility; the mental health professions can support and sympathize, but cannot change what nature has dictated. It safely distances the problem from closer and more detailed perusal that could carry with it some uncomfortable challenges. Questions relating to the position of women in a patriarchal society become irrelevant, and the real life experiences and situations of women can easily be brushed away. Anti-depressants and 'minor' tranquillizers, the latter now known to have some rather 'major' long-term consequences, have commonly been prescribed to sad, unhappy and anxious women. Certainly, in one respect, the drug companies and the medical profession have got it right, since medication can reduce symptoms, but it does not address the question of why is there such a high incidence of depression among women, and why it continues to grow.

The hormonal explanation is reflected most obviously in the myth of the depressed, menopausal middle-aged woman, and it is a powerful and familiar argument. But it is a myth. Reid and Yen[4] have convincingly demonstrated that there is no evidence of increased risk of depression during the menopause, and else-where[5] it has, in addition, been shown that only about 10 per cent of women have any feelings of regret about the cessation of periods.

In many ways these findings are surprising. Cultural stereo-types powerfully present the desirability for women of eternal youth; a visitor from outer space, scanning our television programmes and the popular press, could be forgiven for thinking that women remained permanently aged twenty-five.

The advertising industry is an influential one and its messages are far-reaching. The underlying stereotypes, and their demoralizing effect on women, should not be underestimated. Typically, women are presented in one of two ways. They are either portrayed as young, slim and sexual, or, in Courtney and Whipple's words:

> She [woman] is shown as a housewife and mother dependent upon male authority for her decisions. She is shown as desperately in need of product benefits to satisfy and serve her husband and family, and it is from this service that she draws her self-esteem. In addition, she has a pressing need for personal adornment to help her attract and hold a man.[6]

They also note that the 'absence of older and minority group women from advertising [makes] them an invisible part of society'. This is not the case with men. Older men, for example, are depicted as responsible, dignified, and authoritative. Neither are they viewed as unattractive; and are often seen in the company of young and beautiful women, who apparently hang on to their every word. A younger woman attached to an older man is seen as glamorous and acceptable. The converse is not true for women; a younger man attached to an older woman may be described as a 'toy boy' or 'gigolo', and the woman accused of 'cradle-snatching'. In popular jargon, men 'mature' and women 'grow old'.

It is, therefore, perhaps surprising that the rate of depression among middle-aged women, although rising, is not higher than it is. To be part of a society that rates youth so highly, that allows men as they grow older to do so with a status and a dignity, and without loss of perceived sexual attractiveness, while simultaneously denying such rights to women, does indeed pose dilemmas. Although some women experience depression as a result of such difficulties, the fact that more do not is a matter of surprise, and is a tribute to the extraordinary strength and resilience of women. Perhaps women are aware that although the menopause can indeed be a trying time, they are well used to trials, and surviving them, by that point in their lives. Although popular culture and mythology may dictate that the menopause is somehow the Rubicon in the life of a woman, she may know differently.

So why do women get depressed? Ask this question of any group of women, and the answer will invariably, and not facetiously, be 'men!' It is frequently followed by general surprise that the rate of depression is no higher than it is. Obviously such a stark and brief answer requires further expansion and enquiry, but the universality and spontaneity of the response is noteworthy. In expanding on their answer, I refer to what women themselves say.

Why women get depressed

Taking responsibility

Women feel that they take on responsibility for relationships. This is in itself a huge task, but when relationships break down, women tend to see it as their own fault. They will all too often say 'What did I do wrong?' or 'What wasn't I able to give?', rather than 'He has a problem maintaining and making relationships', or, 'It didn't work for us'. Given that we are living in a society where a third of marriages end in divorce, and others struggle along unhappily, this involves a huge pool of unhappy relationships. In this pool it frequently seems to be the woman who is left floundering to keep herself afloat, while simultaneously trying to stop others from drowning, particularly children. If, at the same time, she sees herself as responsible for entering such dangerous waters, and blames herself for not having foreseen their murky depths, she is likely to experience enormous psychological stresses.

Self via another

Additionally, women themselves feel that they fall into the trap of securing their own identity via their relationships, primarily as wife or partner to a man, but also through motherhood, and through being a daughter. It should not be forgotten that considerable numbers of elderly parents are cared for by their daughters. Far fewer are cared for by their sons; their place is, of course, in the world outside the home. Similarly, about 90 per cent of single parents are mothers (although more fathers are now joining their ranks). Small children are still mainly cared for by their mothers, or by female substitutes. Women are the carers, but who cares for them? As we shall come to see, caring is a role that society may pay lip-service to, but does not back up with provision of adequate resources.

If we accept that a woman's identity is frequently gained through another, it follows that if the other, in any sense, ceases to be, a large part of her sense of self and of self-worth is liable to tumble. The study by Brown and Harris that suggests that work is a protector against depression would fit into this model. Work not only gives women some financial independence and status, (important in this strongly capitalist society) but also gives them another source of validity, another route to a sense of self that is not tied up so directly with being responsible for, and defined through, another person. The protective aspect of employment is very clearly felt and expressed by women.

Placing value on relationships

Women themselves feel that they give more to their relationships than men, and thus have more to lose. They feel that they make a real commitment and perhaps are able to relate more easily at a deeper and essentially different level. Perhaps they are more prepared to take risks for what they see as valuable and significant, but they can also interpret this in themselves as being 'naive', 'stupid', or 'unrealistic'. It may be that women essentially place more value on relating and being than on doing and profit-making. It would certainly appear that from a young age (as we have seen in an earlier chapter) boys are encouraged outwards into the world, whereas girls are drawn inwards. Women's feelings of responsibility for relationships, together with their real lack of power in the wider world, leave them feeling as if they are walking a tight rope in a high wind without a safety net. Dorothy Dinnerstein suggests that woman

> thus carries the moral obligations of the parent while suffering the powerlessness of the child. Man, conversely, carries parental power while enjoying the child's freedom from moral obligation. He has the right, like the child, to remain unaware of, uninterested in, [woman's] point of view . . . this means that he is encouraged in a kind of moral laziness which stunts his growth: his capacities for empathetic emotional generosity atrophy through disuse.[7]

Expectations versus realities

Young women, then, may face a huge shock as they enter the world; they find that what they have been encouraged to do, and how they have been brought up to be, is out of tune with what the wider world demands, expects and rewards. Women see themselves as having been brought up to care; they are also brought up to believe that their future lies with men, who will in turn care for and protect them. The latter may turn out to be a false expectation, and the former an unrewarded and unsupported way of life.

Do young women really expect relationships with men to provide love and security? Jacqueline Sarsby[8] found that teenage girls emphasize security and having a man to support them as reasons for marrying. They also want to be needed; to be especially important to someone. They express their needs consistently in financial and emotional terms. Men's needs are more practical and domestic, with emotional needs not so paramount. This represents a considerable gap in expectations, in a world that is already characterized by lack of equality of opportunity between men and women. It could be argued that one disappointment after another awaits women as they become adult, particularly for young working-class women who are less likely to gain access to higher education and careers. Liz Heron suggests that:

> Tinsel romance sustains us and betrays us, a tantalising mockery of longing, yet never to be despised for the longings and desires it expresses. In the pulp romance of everyday, romance rewards femininity with symbiosis: the illusory security of the womb, the regained safety of arms that encircle and hold close, the bliss of merging with another. But in offering to women the lure of protection, the easy abdication of responsibility, it fashions an unequal symbiosis.[9]

The myth of marriage

Is marriage somehow a lure, a false promise of security and protection? For many of the depressed women interviewed by Brown and Harris it was certainly true that marriage had not given them the closeness and security they had hoped for. This is backed up consistently by other research findings, for example in studies by Gove,[10] Gove and Tudor,[11] and Bachrach[12] all of which conclude that marriage has a protective role for men, but a detrimental effect on women, in terms of their mental health. Catherine Itzin, suggests that even given the hardships and anxieties experienced by single mothers, 'these single parent people are – without exception – happier as single parents than they were married, even [those who were] "happily" married'.[13] This pattern was also evident in the women interviewed by Sue Sharpe. Such findings might appear somewhat surprising as they are in sharp contradiction to popularly held, and media-reinforced, mythology.

This myth of the protection of marriage at least in part explains the class differential in depression among women. Middle-class girls are still far more likely to enter higher education and the professions; they are more likely to marry and have children as a positive choice, rather than as the only route into adulthood.

Having had children, they are more likely to remain in or return promptly to work. If they stay at home with young children this can be seen as an interim measure and the exercise of choice. Although they still face the risk of depression, the risk is smaller.

Since employment may be a real protection against depression, and educated, middle-class women do have easier access to work, and indeed to higher-paid work, this may make life somewhat easier for them. But they, too, have their own conflicts and confusions, as we saw with Suzanne in Chapter 1. Ability and apparent success may not be an insulation against very severe unhappiness. Social background cannot protect against family difficulty or disaster; it does not remove societal pressures and psychologically imposed barriers, although it can open more doors when psychological difficulties are overcome. Perhaps the analogy is that there are somewhat fewer fronts to have to fight the battle on. Easier access to education, and relatively well-paid jobs thereafter, should not be underestimated in their protective value.

Children: contradictions and conflicts

When discussing the causes of depression with women, the subject of children inevitably, though anxiously, arises. The implications of motherhood were considered in some detail in Chapter 5, but it has a particular relevance when examining women and depression. Most women have children; and most girls are brought up to see this as part of their future destiny. Motherhood carries with it a status of its own, and for women with little access to any other status this can be a very real pull. At last you are someone – you are a mother. The reasons for having a child can be complex. Pregnancy can be carefully planned, or a total surprise – pleasant or otherwise. It can be an attempt to gain a sense of completeness. It can be a means of cementing or formalizing a relationship. It can be a statement of identity or an attempt to discover one. It can be a functional decision in terms of an overall life plan, a natural progression at a particular stage of life. Whatever it is about, and however it is understood, after the birth of a child life will never be the same again for a woman. She will experience agonies and ecstasies that are difficult to comprehend beforehand.

The intensity of feelings, and the contradictory nature of many of these, are familiar to all mothers. It certainly appears that life at home with children makes many women susceptible to depression. Why is this? Certainly, the birth of a child, and the reality of the ongoing daily (and nightly) care can be very different from the smiling madonna image of pregnancy. The first three months of a baby's life can be particularly difficult, and Sheila Kitzinger[14] argues for far greater awareness of this as a particularly vulnerable time. As children grow older, their demands and needs change and develop, and the person who cares for them (still most often primarily the mother, especially in the early years) has to have both internal and external resources if these needs are to be adequately met. The internal and external resources inevitably overlap and interrelate. But without sufficient external resources it is difficult to see how the internal strengths needed for caring for children can be nurtured and developed.

Let us look at the reality of childcare in the UK. It has already been suggested that motherhood carries some status, but it is, in reality, a nominal status. It is not backed by economic status, and in British society, which is powerfully capitalist and patriarchal it therefore carries little weight. On the one hand, mothers are told they are doing a valuable job; on the other hand, little provision or payment is made to validate this message. However much mothers love their children, this cannot be translated into ongoing and happy care if they themselves feel isolated, alone, devalued and unsupported. Depression is the all too frequent result, and many children grow up in an impoverished and depressing environment. As Sue Sharpe states:

> What is under attack is the hypocritical way in which the importance of motherhood and parenting in general is underestimated. Motherhood is idealized yet it is given a very low status and minimal social provision and this is reflected in the conditions under which mothers bear children and subsequently care for them. At present, mothering, and especially full time mothering at home, often takes place in conditions that amount to severe social deprivation where women may be cut off from other adults, from outside interests, from adult conversation and other stimulation, and are potentially vulnerable to depression and other psychological disorders.[15]

Whether the current and growing need to attract women back into the labour market will bring about a sudden mushrooming in childcare facilities, as it has in the past, is doubtful. The UK may continue with its dubious reputation of having almost the worst childcare provision in Europe.[16] It is notable that only 44 per cent of our three- to five-year-olds are in public pre-school education, the second lowest percentage in the EC. The provision for 0–2-

year-olds is even worse, and caters for only 2 per cent of this age group. Again, this is almost the worst in the EC, with only Luxembourg and Ireland lagging even further behind. Yet again this affects working-class mothers to a greater extent than middle-class mothers. The latter group, because of their higher earning potential, and because their hours of work are likely to be less rigid, have more access to private sector provision.

Surely if childcare and mothering are of such vital significance (and obviously they are), then mothers and their children deserve more and better. They do not deserve to be fed platitudes, myths and false images of what cannot be attained. They deserve facilities and resources that respond to their real needs, which would enable women to make a choice. That choice is essentially one that would enable women either to care for their own children in their own home or to remain in the labour market if they so wish. For there to be a real choice, both options need the backing of resources and a firm commitment to women and their children. If this does not happen the worrying findings of the Brown and Harris study will not change.

For many women the balancing act of caring for children, caring for their relationship, looking after a home, and being in employment, is a stressful and demanding one. This was summed up by Jane, a woman who had recently returned to work. She had received psychiatric out-patient care for depression and then been referred for counselling:

> I got home the other night and I was so tired. And everyone wanted something. And I wanted to say go away and leave me alone. But I felt so guilty. And I thought, it doesn't work. I should really just stay at home. I just can't be everything to all people all of the time. But before I went back to work I got really fed up so I don't know what to do. I sometimes feel there is a great big hole in me, an emptiness waiting to be filled up. And then my mother rang me to ask me if I'd made my jam yet. Well! She's got no idea. And she says I should work if I want to. Then she'll say: 'Of course I could never have left you with a stranger. I'd have worried and you would have hated it.' And it makes me feel so angry and so guilty. And then, my husband will help, but I have to ask him, just like asking the children. Why can't he just clean the kitchen without asking – if it's obvious to me it must be obvious to him. I thought of leaving him once but I was horrified. I thought, oh no, I couldn't leave him, I just wouldn't feel whole.

As the reader will see, the conflicts for this woman were many and complex. In considering the process of counselling and therapy with women who are depressed, the way Jane began to resolve these issues will be discussed.

The experience of loss

Brown and Harris suggest that depression is often triggered by some form of loss. In their study, they focus on some key factors in provoking depression: the experience of loss or disappointment; the threat of separation, or actual separation, from a key person; a major financial loss; and unpleasant news regarding someone close. Remembering that they also identified the significance of the childhood loss of a mother, it is worth noting that the losses of today may well recreate or be intensified by losses of the past, especially those that lie unrecognized or unresolved. The question of loss of mother, identified in a literal sense by Brown and Harris, may involve other aspects, which I return to below.

If loss is accepted as a cause of depression, it is important to question whether women experience more losses than men, and if so, what might be the nature of these losses. Many women seem to feel that they do experience more losses than men. Childbirth, for example, may be portrayed through a rose-coloured haze, but in actuality may be experienced through a cloud of depression and exhaustion. Many women experience the actual birth as a profound separation and loss, but this psychological and physiological experience is accompanied by other losses. Many women give up their jobs, and with them financial independence and status. They can lose the basis of their previous relationship with their partner, and often miss the social contact that is a central part of work. Their world shrinks in size and scope, and choices can feel very limited.

As we saw in Chapter 5, the experience of pregnancy itself is not straightforward for many women. Miscarriages are not always viewed with much concern by others but can be devastating for the woman concerned, and stillbirth even more so. Abortion may be the only resolution in other circumstances, but is a loss that will pursue some women for many years, often unrecognized by those around them. The inability to have children, or even a decision not to do so, can be alienating in a world that assumes this to be a natural role.

The times when children start school, become adolescent, leave home, and marry, can be difficult for some mothers, particularly when their central role has been as carer for their children. Re-entering the labour market can be problematic; years of caring for children are not given much credence by employers, and women themselves are very aware that men have risen in power and status. This gap is very hard to bridge, and the earlier losses relating to employment when a family is first started, are again placed under the spotlight.

Rape and violent assault, as we shall see in Chapter 8, are experienced as the most appalling invasion of the body and the self, and result in women feeling they have lost an essential part of their own being. At the time it feels an irrevocable loss, and recovery can be a very slow process. Abuse in childhood, sexual harassment in adulthood, lead to feelings of loss of part of the self; as well as loss of hope, and loss of trust.

Other losses may be less obvious, but nevertheless are significant. Having themselves given up their place in the labour market, or having compromised with part-time work or less satisfying and demanding work, many women then face a further adjustment. Their partner's job may require moving home if he is to progress. Traditionally women have followed their men, but frequently have to leave behind friends and homes to which they have become attached. This can have a very special significance not appreciated by male partners, who has not been part of the world of women, having been busily occupied in another.

I referred earlier to the significance of the death of the mother in childhood. The trauma of this is obvious. There are, however, other aspects of losing a mother that need recognition. It may be that mothers have a more ambivalent relationship towards their daughters, both wanting them to be different from them but, at the same time, like them. Mothers may, therefore, in some senses, give daughters less, or give them more confusing messages, than they give their sons. This can result in a sense of loss of identity, and of uncertainty about the self, and additionally as Eichenbaum and Orbach suggest:

> A girl grows up learning she will have to give up her mother without getting wifely love in its place. Paradoxically, precisely because men have the continuity that women are denied, male needs are less exposed.[17]

The list is long. It needs to be seen in the context of a world in which women are often aware of the inherent losses that are a result of the inequality in Western society. The very fact of their gender implies lost or unavailable opportunities. Arieti and Bemporad make this point well:

> Depressed women are more likely to mourn not of the castration of their penis, which would be pure fantasy on their part, but because they really have been castrated – although in a metaphorical sense. The symbolic penis of which they have been deprived is the male role in the world.[18]

It seems that the losses experienced by women are many, and that they operate on many levels. However, it is equally evident that the creation and maintenance of at least some of the loss-producing situations is a direct result of society organizing itself in such a way as to diminish the opportunities of women to be themselves.

An alternative rage

Traditional notions of femininity paint a picture of women who are gentle, caring, submissive and peaceable. The expression of anger is not part of the stereotype; indeed, it is seen as non-feminine. Yet women have much to be angry about, but, because of the power of the stereotype, often have considerable difficulty in expressing it. One might reasonably expect that those in the business of caring for women are sufficiently aware of the dangers of stereotyping that they take care not to reinforce these images, but work with women to enable free expression and acceptance of all their feelings, including anger. Unfortunately, studies have shown that this is not the case. The study by Broverman and her colleagues[19], that I have referred to elsewhere, examined the attitudes of mental health professionals to men and women. They examined how this group defined a mentally healthy adult, and compared this to definitions of mentally healthy men and women.

This study confirms that those involved in mental health care *are* caught up in stereotyping. It is worrying that those who care for women when they are at their most vulnerable and distressed should hold these attitudes. Broverman and her colleagues demonstrate that to be seen as mentally healthy, women have to suppress the qualities of anger, assertiveness and independence that make for a healthy adult. Men on the other hand, do not. The definition of a healthy man corresponds to that of a healthy adult. This discrepancy gives considerable cause for concern. It is again made clear that the expression of anger in women is not acceptable. It can even be seen as a symptom of mental ill health in women (though not in men).

Small wonder that women have so much difficulty in explicitly expressing anger. But it has to go somewhere. In a society that denies the outward expression of anger to women, they have no choice but to bury it deep within themselves. Anger, when buried and repressed, turns to depression, and acknowledging this with women helps them to uncover and explore their anger.

Working with depressed women: the process of therapy and counselling

Getting near

> One of the worst things for me when I'm really depressed is when people try and keep me at arm's length. I can't get near them, and they won't get near me. And the other awful thing is when someone pretends that it's just a bad day and tries to jolly me out of it. Because it's just not like that when you're really depressed.

This awful sense of isolation which Anne describes is frequently encountered by counsellors and therapists working with depressed women. Such is the hopelessness of the client that the counsellor may also feel that s/he can make no contact and can be of no use in the face of overwhelming despair. Perhaps, as Anne describes, this may precipitate a weary helper into removing herself/himself to a safe distance, or alternatively into exhibiting false and entirely unhelpful cheeriness. It can also be that the client has mixed feelings about letting anyone near: depression often involves an uncomfortable mix of wanting someone to take it all away and believing that no one can do anything (and in any case would not want to). A male counsellor has to be especially careful not to fall into the category of the powerful oppressor who cannot possibly understand anyway, while a female counsellor can become simply another suffering victim, as oppressed and depressed and helpless as her client.

Throughout counselling and therapy the ability to stay near a woman in her depression, without being sucked into the experience, is essential. Depression is frightening; helpers who distance themselves may suggest that they are frightened, too. I will return to Anne later to see what she herself said about this, but first we need to see how her counsellor responded to her. As these words came in an early session it seemed important to find out from Anne just how much support was available to her in her own world.

In fact she had little at the time of therapy, and additionally she came from a family in which, as the oldest child and only daughter, she had been expected to take on a caring role from a very early age, also acting as a mediator between fighting parents. As she grew older she repeated this pattern: she gathered around her those in need of care and support as a way of re-affirming her rather shaky sense of self. Entering her first adult relationship was for a while a joyous experience, but as her own needs started to emerge and were expressed, that relationship ended. Neither her friends nor her family were able to cope with the resulting unhappy and needy Anne that emerged.

From this early information several significant strands of her life emerged that had implications for the therapist's relationship with Anne. While the immediate trigger for her depression was undoubtedly the ending of an important relationship, dealing with it on that level alone would not have been sufficient. What was uncovered was a lifetime of having to care for others, and of meeting others' needs, with the accompanying feeling that this was the only safe and acceptable way to be. A new relationship had given the hope of something different, but this hope was cruelly dashed. It gradually became apparent that yet again she was with someone who was in love with her coping persona, but not with her whole self. The reaction of others to her distress then served again to confirm what she had always felt: to be acceptable she must be loving, caring and supportive. To receive acceptance for herself she had first to fulfil – and to go on fulfilling – that role. This extended to her being in a caring role in her working life.

It was very important that her female therapist acknowledged Anne's fear that she (her therapist) would be unable to cope with her neediness and unhappiness, and would then distance herself in the same way that others had done. It was also important to reassure Anne that this would not be the case, although this was a reassurance that was tested time after time, and that had to be given repeatedly. In acknowledging this fear it was also important for Anne to begin to understand how this had arisen for her: that her fear related not just to recent events but that it had a long history.

It might reasonably be asked how therapists and counsellors demonstrate to someone that they are staying near, and not likely to retreat to a safe inaccessible distance. The quality of nearness to someone – in any context – is a difficult one to describe, although it seems that clients are very good at identifying its absence or presence, as are others in different relationships.

Getting near does not mean identifying yourself with the other. Comments such as 'I know just how you feel, I went through exactly the same thing myself' are not only presumptuous, they may be quite inaccurate and detract from allowing a woman to tell her own story in her own time. Neither is it helpful to try and rescue someone from their depression by making false promises – 'We'll soon have you better, dear, just take these for a few weeks. It's really nothing to worry about, lots of women your age go through this' – typical of the type of bland reassurance offered to many women. There are counselling equivalents to the medical magic of the prescription pad that do not allow autonomy and exploration, but impose programmes and suggest strategies. They may have a part to play, but used alone they cannot touch the complexities of depression. They carry with them the danger of oversimplifying the nature of the experience of not allowing the pain to be expressed, and of distancing the counsellor from the client.

Working with Anne, her therapist showed how she could 'stay near' in a number of ways. Both initially, and over the period of the year in therapy, it was important to reassure Anne that the relationship was not dependent on her presenting her competent and caring persona. Anne needed to discover that her therapist would stay with her throughout, that her therapist would survive the distress, the anger, the demands, the neediness, and the pain that were all to be expressed. Not only would she survive, she would not be damaged, and would enable Anne to express these feelings, and to start to make sense of them. In that way a part of Anne that she feared and associated with rejection, was accepted both by her therapist and then by herself. Her therapist was not frightened, and did not reject. The time came when her acceptance of Anne enabled Anne to accept herself. At the end of therapy, when Anne and her therapist were looking back together over the course of the year, Anne herself put it this way:

> You made me feel safe and you never ran away from how bad I was feeling, even when I wished I could myself, I felt so bad. And sometimes I wanted to push you away, and I really did push as hard as I could, just so I could say to myself, there, she's just like all the others. But you didn't go away, you'd always be there when you said

you would, and sometimes I couldn't believe it. But you weren't just a sponge either, you weren't just passive. You'd put things back to me; you'd check things out; you'd try and make sense of it all. It sounds simple, but that feeling that I've never managed to frighten you away, even when I wanted just to die, has really mattered. Somehow I felt you really got close to *me* and that mattered.

So perhaps the quality of being near can be defined after all – it is the ability of the counsellor or therapist to really be there, and to stay there. But what does that mean? It means being available, without being invasive; being accepting and listening, without falling into bland reassurance or false agreement; being challenging, without being threatening; and not abandoning the client when she encounters herself at her bleakest. In depression women often feel inaccessible to themselves, let alone others, and it is crucial that the therapist is able to tolerate their experiences and feelings, however awful they seem. Some descriptions of depression vividly portray the bleakness of that experience:

It's like being trapped inside a glass capsule. It's narrow and soundproofed. You can see, but can't touch, and can't hear. You are trapped inside, and others are trapped and unattainable outside.

It's a state of non-being.

It's like being on the end of a long rope, swinging around and around. It's quite pointless. But there's no way of getting off. And it's too far to jump to the ground.

A straightjacket around my heart.

Like being in a grey fog.

These descriptions make it obvious how intense the isolation can be. In a therapeutic relationship, as in any other, the participation of more than one person is needed. Given that depression makes participation hard for the client involved, it really is essential that the therapist does not escape into a haze of false reassurances, use questionnaires to assess the level of depression, make clever interpretations, or create behavioural programmes. Any of these may help the therapist or counsellor feel reassured and quite clever, and even perhaps a little superior. It may demonstrate that s/he has special skills which the client apparently does not have. But, manifested in this way, their value must be questioned. Any need to use skills in this quasi-powerful way suggests that counsellors and therapists might need to look at themselves. Skills have become a substitute for the use of oneself.

They may be valuable, but doing cannot replace being. Doing things may feel safer, more controllable, and more comfortable, but it does not enable exploration of the experience of depression.

Safety nets and lifelines

The images of depression quoted above suggest that one aspect of depression is the feeling of being powerless and out of control. This experience of life carrying on regardless, and without one's permission, is very disturbing. I have argued that 'doing' often precludes being, exploring, and making sense of the world; nevertheless, when someone is seriously depressed, and worried that they may not be able to continue functioning, it *is* useful to explore with them whether they can find safety nets and lifelines. Counsellors need to remind themselves that there are sometimes practical solutions to practical problems. Also, finding something or someone that will catch you, or hold on to you, or allow you to hold on, in your bleakest or most difficult moments can literally be a lifesaver. The value of this should not be underestimated. Such added support can make the process of working with a depressed woman less anxiety-provoking for both parties. It can ease and speed the process.

But it is of crucial importance that such systems of help and support are explored with the client. Exploration and encouragement should not give way to imposing demands and solutions, either implicitly or explicitly. It may be helpful to look at those times and situations in a woman's life that feel hardest to cope with, and then to look with her at how she feels they could become more tolerable. This helps reduce the feeling of being over-whelmed by the enormity of it all, and she may well find ways of gaining some control over some aspects of it. When your world has become apparently uncontrollable, that in itself can be reassuring.

However, it must be the client, and not the counsellor, who is exerting control. Women often feel they have little control over their lives and this is reflected in the reality of their experiences. The counsellor must be very careful not to reinforce this feeling. Enabling a woman to start taking charge of her life, while working with her on other past and present issues, is very different to issuing instructions as to what she should do in order to feel better. One young depressed mother recalled a male psychiatrist telling her that she should get her mother to help with the children at bedtimes. She was sent off with a cheerful 'Now you do that, and that will make things much easier for you'. The following week when she had failed to follow the instruction, she was met with the veiled threat: 'Now we can't help you if you won't help yourself can we?' The assumptions and stereotypes contained in that interaction are obvious. What the psychiatrist did not know, and did not attempt to find out, was that the young woman had a very poor relationship with her mother, and was struggling to separate from her. She could not ask her mother, nor was it desirable that she should do so.

Sometimes there is no support available, or none that can be identified or experienced, especially when depression is very severe. Anne appeared to have none when she said:

> There is no one I can turn to; no one who helps. No one wants me when I'm like this. I'm totally alone. Nothing I do helps. I just feel awful all the time.

When someone feels this way, and expresses it so absolutely, accepting the reality as described by that person, while not yourself falling into the pit of despair, can be difficult. Starting to unravel the tangle of experiences and feelings that result in this unhappiness is not straightforward. But the knot can sometimes be eased so it allows room for the woman to move, when previously she felt in a strait-jacket. This was so for Anne. For some while nobody and nothing lifted the weight of deeply oppressive feelings. Gradually, as work progressed with her, she was able to let other people in. She began, very tentatively, to test her acceptability to others when she was feeling unhappy. She began to see that she had perhaps selected needy friends. After all, her caring persona was a safe one for her, and gave her a sense of identity. It was a breakthrough for her, when she was feeling very unhappy, to be able to ring a friend. She said afterwards:

> She couldn't take it all away, or do anything, but she did listen, and she did care, and said I was silly not to tell her before. She rang me the next night to see how I was.

From this point on, Anne was able to find some lifelines. She could not have done this sooner. Imposing suggestions on her would not have worked. She could only do this when she had some understanding of why it was so difficult for her to rely on others, and when she began to feel safe enough within the therapeutic relationship to be able tentatively to make moves outside it.

No magic wands and no instant cures

As we have seen, women are usually depressed for very good reasons. Depression does not magically disappear overnight, and it would be failing to take either the causes or the experience seriously, for a therapist to give false hopes that all will suddenly be well. In fact, starting to talk about experiences and feelings effectively lifts the lid off a lot that has been repressed. Inevitably, while this can be a great relief, it can also be painful. But it does not produce instantaneous recovery. Conflict and real difficulties may be exposed which can result in major decisions or compromises having to be made.

It can be helpful if this is explained to the client. As we have seen, taking charge of herself, and control over her own life, can be an important part of starting to deal with depression. The other side of the coin is perhaps that therapists and counsellors need to share honestly and openly with their women clients their understanding of the process. Too often women are treated as passive recipients of various forms of treatment, when they should be as actively involved as possible, and know what it is they are choosing to do.

What I mean, of course, is not that depressed women should passively and resignedly accept their depression, but rather that they should be made aware that the resolution of depression is not something that can be done *to* them. It involves two people working together as honestly as possible; while this might at times be painful, it also carries with it hope. It can be easier for women if they are not too frightened by their depression; as we have seen, fright is generally a response that is comprehensible and hardly surprising. Because it does not go instantly, and has to be lived with for a while, therapy needs to be seen as an ongoing process and not as the magic wand that makes everything better. But not only is it good to be rid of magic wands because they are mythical; it is also vital that therapy is not seen as an incomprehensible, magic process, since this robs women of the control they so much need to take.

Exploring the conflicts

Perhaps what is really needed is an approach that takes real account of women's experiences and the conflicts they feel, and that gives validity to these, enabling women to start making sense of their own lives. Hannah, recently divorced with three children, neatly encapsulates the problem experienced by many:

> Everyone keeps telling me to do my own thing; to assert my rights; to do what I want. How can I? And if I do, what about the children? Doing what I want just doesn't match up with what they need. And if anything goes wrong with them I'll be blamed.

Her situation is not unusual:

> I don't know how to be any more. I mean, what is normal? He's gone, and lives with ever such a young woman. If I found a young man it would be viewed as vaguely obscene, not as glamorous and adventurous. It's always different for women isn't it? How could I just have someone move in here, even if just for a few days for a bit of fun? I mean, with three children, can you imagine it? And my mother says, oh, you can't have men around, not with the children in the house. Well, they're always in the bloody house. It feels impossible. I wish I was dead quite often. He'd have to look after them then. I'm a lousy mother anyway. How can you not be when you're this depressed?

The conflicts are on so many levels that unravelling them and identifying them is complex. How to cope with the demands of a relationship, or how to incorporate potential new relationships into an existing family structure? Is it possible to meet your own needs, or will this inevitably be at the expense of someone else? What, if anything, should you expect from men? Is it possible to lead a fulfilled life without a man? Will there be any support from anyone else? Women in this position are, in addition, very tired. They cope with a long day, many demands, and often have little support.

How do we start to work with these kinds of dilemma, which occur so frequently, in the process of counselling women? Attempting to unravel the individual dynamics from the realities and practicalities, the imposed structures from the needlessly absorbed and the unintentionally maintained, and the responses to the present from hangovers from the past, is not an easy task. For many women, clarification opens up choices. Jane, for instance, decided that she was not prepared to carry all the caring in the family, and the resulting guilt when she was unable constantly and totally to respond. She began to feel that even if the risk did not pay off, and the marriage ended, she would be able to survive and grow in her own right. In fact, after a stormy period, the relationship continued on a changed footing. Jane's depression lifted, and she seemed to have found a much firmer and more solid sense of self. And when her mother next asked whether she had made jam, she replied that she had not had time, but would be delighted to have some of her mother's! This answer apparently pleased both of them, perhaps because it gave validity to both worlds, and united rather than divided them.

Hannah found a different solution. The picture was more fragmented for her. Her mourning for her lost relationship with her husband was long. Issues relating to the expression of her sexuality continued to trouble her. Not only were there difficulties to do with what was and was not acceptable behaviour, but she also felt that the only way to prove her feminine identity was always to have a sexual partner. Her serious depressions in the past had always been related to losses or separations, and her reactions had always been severe. Work with her over a long period finally uncovered very early abuse, known to her family, although the perpetrator had not been a family member.

It was not until that stage that any improvement occurred, and even then it was slow and painful. With Hannah, it would have been very easy to understand her depression purely in terms that related to her current position, which was indeed unenviable. That would have been a mistake. Care has always to be taken not to jump to rapid and oversimplified conclusions. Jane began to be able to make moves and choices when the way was sufficiently clear. Hannah's difficulties had a different origin, and clearing the way with her was more problematic. The current conflicts and difficulties she experienced were real. But there were other layers that had to be uncovered.

The rising rate of depression among women is a serious and worrying problem. It is neither acceptable nor accurate to see depression simply as an individual dysfunction. Treatment, if it is to be effective and not oppressive, should not reflect that stance. Those working with depressed women need to be fully aware of the role of social structures and the socialization of women, and the effects of these in creating and maintaining depression in women. The difficulties facing women in their daily lives must be addressed, and it is essential that the reality of these difficulties is actively acknowledged in therapy and counselling. There is a need for wider social and political awareness among medical and mental health professionals. Outdated and unsubstantiated theories relating to women and depression must be re-examined carefully. Many of them should be dismissed altogether.

Notes

1 Brown, G. and Harris, T. (1978). *Social Origins of Depression*. Tavistock.

2 Richman, N. (1976). 'Depression in mothers of preschool children', *Journal of Child Psychology and Psychiatry*, 17, pp. 75–8.

3 Sharpe, S. (1984). *Double Identity, The Lives of Working Mothers*. Penguin, p. 80.

4 Reid, R.L. and Yen, S.S.C. (1981). 'Premenstrual syndrome', *American Journal of Obstetric Gynaecology*, 139, 1, pp. 85–104.

5 Friedman, R.C. (ed.) (1982). *Behavior and the Menstrual Cycle*. New York: Marcel Dekker.

6 Courtney, A. and Whipple, T. (1980). *Sex Stereotyping in Advertising*. Lexington Books, p. 24.

7 Dinnerstein, D. (1987). *The Rocking of the Cradle and the Ruling of the World*. The Women's Press, p. 236.

8 Sarsby, J. (1983). *Romantic Love and Security*. Penguin.

9 Heron, L. (1986). *Changes of Heart: Reflections on Women's Independence*. Pandora Press, p. 131.

10 Gove, W.R. (1972). 'The relationship between sex roles, marital status and mental illness', *Social Forces*, 51, pp. 34–44.

11 Gove, W.R. and Tudor, F.J. (1973). 'Sex, marital status, and morality', *Americal Journal of Sociology*, 79, pp. 45–67.

12 Bachrach, L. (1975). 'Marital status and mental disorder', *Analytic Review Publication*, 75–217, Washington, D.C.: Dept. of Health, Education and Welfare.

13 Itzin, C. (1980). *Splitting Up*. Virago.

14 Kitzinger, S. (1975). 'The fourth trimester', *Midwife, Health Visitor and Community Nurse*, 11, pp. 118–21.

15 Sharpe, *Double Identity*, pp. 39–40.

16 Figures quoted are from *Labour Review* (March 1989), using source material from Moss, P. *Consolidated Report to the European Commission* (April 1988).

17 Eichenbaum, L. and Orbach, S. (1983). *What Do Women Want?* Michael Joseph, p. 18.

18 Arieti, S. and Bemporad, J. (1978). *Severe and Mild Depression: The Psychotherapeutic Approach*. New York: Basic Books, p. 368.

19 Broverman, I., Broverman, D., Clarkson, F., Rosenkrantz, P. and Vogel, S. (1970). 'Sex role stereotypes and clinical judgements of mental health', *Journal of Consulting and Clinical Psychology*, 34, 1, pp. 1–7.

7

Eating disorders: women, food, and the world

What is the matter with Mary Jane?
She's crying with all her might and main,
And she won't eat her dinner – rice pudding again –
What is the matter with Mary Jane?

A.A. Milne

To attempt to understand eating disorders, and their significance for women, can be a messy task. It can seem a tangle of extraordinary complexity, and starting to examine the resulting muddle induces feelings of simultaneous fascination and dislike. Even writing about the subject reflects something of the experience of women who have difficulties with food. I find myself developing a love/hate relationship towards the subject. I cannot leave it alone. I am intrigued with it. I know I want to write about it. But at the same time I am also definite in not wanting to. So I find myself disliking the subject intensely. I would like to ignore it completely. Yet I cannot bear to give it up. I realize that food in the abstract is starting to dominate me. I become unusually aware of food and of the central role it assumes in the everyday life of most women. I realize as I try to write just how often I am interrupted by children, requesting meals for themselves and their assorted friends. I realize that I have to stop three times in the course of one hour to assist in the making of a chocolate cake. I find myself thinking of how much time I spend shopping for and preparing food. I begin to be aware of how easy it would be for food to become the focus for all sorts of conflicts and difficulties.

And I remember a conversation with a client who had a long-term eating disorder. For many years she had had bouts of anorexia, marked by continuous and obsessive thoughts about food, inability to eat, and considerable weight loss. During one particularly tense session with her, when she seemed to disappear deep into herself, I felt both very drawn to her and pushed away by her. She had wanted to come to the session; she did not wish to leave; she wanted me there, but could not let me near. We both seemed to be sinking into a pit of gloom and frustration. I commented that I was feeling like a plate of food; she was both wanting me, but unable to let herself 'feed' from me. If she did allow this, in some way she had to spit me out before I became assimilated. Acknowledging this central conflict eased the tension and we were able to look further at the meaning food held for her. The power of food over this client was considerable; it became all-pervasive in her life, somehow either consuming all her relationships or not allowing them to nourish her.

What is it about food, and consuming it, that makes it such a problem for some women? Food becomes a dominant feature of their lives, although this may manifest itself in different ways and mean different things. Certainly, once one's attention has been caught by food, awareness of it rapidly increases. Those who have lived with someone who is absorbed by food, whether they are on a diet, are training as a chef or dietician, are a fussy, selective child, or indeed an anorexic, will know the tension that can surround mealtimes. A potentially relaxed social occasion rapidly becomes tense. Those present try to say the right things; they attempt to ignore how much, or how little, food is eaten in a situation that can rapidly become an ordeal for all concerned. And mealtimes come around with great regularitiy, and any tension over food gives a situation which is replayed many times over, with increasing intensity.

Families where one member is not eating normally face a genuine dilemma that can rapidly escalate. It is extremely hard to ignore the refusal to eat, and yet confrontation often reinforces the problem. If one reason for not eating is a conscious or unconscious desire to make a statement of some sort, the statement is certainly powerfully made. Refusal to eat is a highly visible way of acting out a statement, regardless of whether or not the individual can verbalize what she wishes to express. Indeed, if it could be said, there would be less need for acting it out. Sometimes, of course, the woman has tried to speak but not been heard. Paradoxically, an effective way of becoming audible and visible, is sometimes to become silent and 'invisible'. One of the ironies of anorexia is that the thinner the anorexic becomes, the more notice is taken of her.

There is, in some respects, a parallel between anorexia in the family and hunger strikes in society. Both are protests: while one is overt and explicitly political, the other may be implicitly so. Anorexia, with its visible thinness, is essentially a political act within the family: it becomes a public statement. Sooner or later others will notice. Politically inspired hunger strikes are accompanied by clear demands and statements. The anorexic may not express these so clearly, but this does not mean that they do not exist. It may simply mean that their expression has been forbidden, ignored, or not recognized. As time goes on, there is a danger that these hidden meanings become so deeply buried, that reaching them is increasingly difficult. The psychological meaning and messages are hidden under layers of obsessive or compulsive behaviour and rituals.

On the other hand, bulimia (excessive eating accompanied by vomiting) is generally secret, and, since a 'normal' weight is generally maintained, it can remain so, hidden successfully from others for years. Although the distinction between anorexia and bulimia seems very obvious, aspects of both can be experienced by the same woman at different times. For both anorexic and bulimic women, life becomes a battleground where food is seen as the enemy. Although this battle with food disguises the real enemy and difficulty, while it is so defined, a woman is on the winning side when she is controlling her food intake and her weight. If her control has slipped she may resort to drastic measures. This is vividly described by one young woman:

> I'd had a really good week. I knew exactly what I'd eaten and exactly how many calories that was. I felt thin, and I felt wonderful. Then it all went. I just stuffed the food into me. I couldn't taste anything or tell you what I'd eaten. I just forced it all down me. Then I had to get rid of it. I can't make myself sick, I just can't do it. So I took over a hundred laxatives.

Her obsession with food, her desire to have absolute control, her failure to maintain this, and her extreme and punitive response to the failure, catch some of the quality of an anorexic's way of life. Food takes over – there is little time to think about anything else. At the same time, food, as every small child knows, can be used to exert powerful pressure.

But why is this such a problem for some women, and why is it mainly women who experience these difficulties with eating? In order to examine this question further, the role of women in relation to food and feeding others needs to be examined in greater detail.

Women, food and the expectations of others

Traditionally, women have taken responsibility for feeding others. It is women who tend to purchase and prepare food for their partners and families. They have a huge range of foods to choose from. In our modern affluent culture, where the majority enjoy relative wealth, food can even be seen as something of a status symbol. The restaurant trade is booming, fast foods are to be found everywhere, and wholefoods and additives have become acceptable topics of conversation. At the same time, the health and exercise cult is much in evidence. Staying fit and being slim have almost become a moral injunction. Disapproval hangs like a cloud over those who despise jogging and dislike low-chloresterol spreads: retribution awaits around the corner.

This is, of course, a far cry from the situation of past generations. The rigours of wartime and post-war rationing are still remembered by many older women. Choice was never an issue; the dilemma was how to nourish a family sufficiently when so little was available. Before the Second World War, incomes were often low and families larger. For many women, feeding hungry mouths meant a combination of anxiety and ingenuity, hours spent in the kitchen, and mothers often going without. Food may indeed have been a major preoccupation, but this was more likely to be related to its scarcity and expense. In those days, food and eating had a functional quality: you ate enough, if you were lucky, to satisfy hunger. It was not a demonstration of sophistication and social standing.

Food leads large numbers of women today into a maze of conflicts and contradictions. They know, as do therapists and counsellors who work with them, that finding the way through the maze is a tortuous and frustrating exercise. Attempting to make sense of the conflicts and contradictions is extremely confusing for all concerned. There is a similar confusion in the way food is presented to women. Magazines are full of delectable recipes, enthusiastically described and gloriously photographed. The hard sell is much in evidence. The implications are twofold: first, that they, too, can cook like this; and second, that to be a real woman they should do so. Yet frequently in the very same magazine there are also slimming diets, often including faintly accusatory statements such as 'How will *you* look in *your* bikini this summer?'. Perhaps the conclusion women reach is that they may cook the food for others, as long as they do not eat it themselves. If they do, they will not be the desired shape and therefore attractive. And in Western society, where women are identified through their bodies, attractiveness is paramount.

Women face an enormous number of demands and expectations, while apparently being offered more with which to meet them. However, these do not always coincide so neatly. Food and eating is one example of the way something is attractively packaged and offered to women while in reality it is not unconditionally available to them. It is the same with the possibility of equal opportunities, of greater access to employment, and other apparent opportunities. The message is: have a little taste but not a great big bite. Do not demand too much, or take too much, or you will pay the price.

It is not only in history and society in this wider sense that food and women are inextricably linked. In an individual's life history this is also the case. Most small children are cared for by the mother, and it is mother who generaly feeds them. For a little girl, it is therefore the same-sex parent who responds to this most basic and essential of needs. Winnicott[1] suggests that the mother's face is a mirror for the baby; that she sees herself and her world reflected there. We have already noted, in looking at women and depression, that there is a high incidence of depression among young women with small children. If the baby girl, when she is being fed, sees mirrored depression and anxiety from the parent she will grow up to be like, a powerful and negative image is present from an early stage.

Although a depressed mother may have very mixed feelings about a child of either sex, there may be some essential differences as to how this ambivalence is experienced towards boy and girl babies. A boy will not grow up to be a woman and a mother. He will belong to a world from which the mother, especially when she has a very young child, is largely excluded. She knows she will have to let go of him to this other male world. A daughter may be viewed very differently. In part, the mother may well wish for more and better access to this larger world for her daughter. But another part wishes her to be like herself, to stay with her, to share the female world. As young babies become small children they very soon become aware of their gender. A girl knows that she is, in some essential ways, like her mother. A boy knows that he is not. What is being suggested is that taking food from a depressed mother, whom in so many ways she will be like, may give a young girl an essentially ambivalent attitude towards both food and the potential or even actual experience of womanhood. While this is particularly clearly so in the case of a depressed mother, it is also relevant to other aspects of the relationship.

The characteristics of eating disorders

Bulimia

Although a distinction has been drawn between anorexia and bulimia, it has also been noted that people can exhibit symptoms of both. My own clinical experience suggests that there is considerable overlap between the two, confirming what has been written elsewhere, with Garfinkel[2] stating that 40 per cent of anorexics become bulimic or move between one and the other.

Mira Dana and Marilyn Lawrence also acknowledge that the relationship between anorexia and bulimia is confusing. They point out that bulimia may be a second stage to anorexia, and, in part, a response to earlier treatment that the younger anorexic may receive. Their argument is a convincing one, related to hospital treatment, commonly used, that emphasizes feeding. The goal of this treatment is clearly defined as reaching a weight that has been defined as appropriate. They point out that achieving weight gain does not tackle underlying psychological issues, and that these remain unresolved. Their research suggests that on discharge from hospital, the weight gain cannot be tolerated, and other methods of weight control are therefore sought. I have known clients who suggest to me that a powerful factor that accompanies this disgust at weight gain is fear of readmission, and more treatment of a similar nature. This may intensify the desire to develop another strategy. Dana and Lawrence describe what a woman can experience on discharge from hospital:

> her loss of control [over food] terrifies her, and she discovers that by vomiting after she has eaten, she can at least control the consequences of her overeating. Such a woman, whose eating disorder goes, as it were, underground, is often regarded by both medical professionals and family as recovered. A normal weight is maintained, a normal seeming life again becomes possible. It is the cost of such normality which remains hidden and a source of such shame.[3]

If anorexia is converted to bulimia in this way, becoming an invisible form of anorexia, it perhaps partially explains the continued popularity of this weight-oriented approach that remains widely used in many hospitals. In the obvious sense, it is successful: weight is gained. Most women at some point have to capitulate to a system that is more powerful than they are. If they are not allowed to get out of bed, not allowed visitors, or not allowed to get dressed until their weight reaches a certain point, the pressure to eat becomes enormous. If after discharge they discover forced vomiting as a technique for dealing both with the weight and the loss of control, they are highly unlikely to reveal this information at follow-up sessions. By not revealing, they re-establish some control for themselves. One round of the battle has been won. At the same time, those treating them will see a successful outcome. A woman in her twenties, who had been hospitalized in her teens for anorexia, describes elements of this experience:

> In the end I had to eat, I wasn't allowed out of bed until I did, and I had a nurse with me all the time at every mealtime. When I left hospital, they were all really pleased with me, because I had reached my target weight. I felt absolutely dreadful. That's when I started bingeing and making myself sick. I couldn't let my weight get too low, because I thought they'd take me back into hospital. But I was taking charge again, and that mattered. I never, ever told the psychiatrist what I was doing. I never told him anything that was going on. I used to feel really triumphant.

Until she was able to refer herself some ten years later this woman lived with a pattern of eating that entirely dominated her life, and at times affected her health. It made the formation of close relationships a great problem, since acknowledging her difficulty to another person was extremely threatening. The underlying causes were complex, and it was evident that her earlier treatment both failed to identify these, and ensured that she would not easily seek help. As Susie Orbach points out, traditional psychiatric responses 'serve to negate her protest. They unwittingly deny the meaning of her symptom and in so doing contribute to its perpetuation. They become part of the problem, rather than part of the solution'.[4]

While it can be argued that behavioural approaches do effectively remove symptoms, other questions need to be asked about such therapy. Being a patient in a hospital can render a usually assertive person passive. If a woman is restricted to bed, is closely supervised, lacks control over her immediate environment, and has few choices, she will be under great pressure to give in to those around her. Those who work in such environments are doubtless well intentioned, but they need to ask if such treatment is either acceptable, or truly effective. Perhaps the words of W.H. Auden deserve some pause for thought:

> Of course behaviourism works. So does torture. Give me a no-nonsense, down to earth behaviorist; a few drugs, and simple electronic appliances, and in six months I will have him reciting the Athanasian creed in public.[5]

Anorexia

Much has been written about the characteristics of anorexia, although what it is, and how it is recognized, tend to be less controversial than trying to unravel what is behind it, and how best to treat it. Hilda Bruch[6] identifies the following signs as typical. Most obviously, there is severe weight loss, accompanied by cessation of periods. Body image becomes distorted, the anorexic seeing herself as fat and overweight, when others are concerned about her thinness and loss of weight. She is unable to recognize her own need for food, can become hyperactive, and unaware of tiredness. She can experience a feeling of effectiveness. Her self-esteem will be very low, and this can be accompanied by powerful feelings of self-hatred and even attempts at suicide. Carried to its conclusion, of course, anorexia leads to death.

Contrary to what one might imagine, the anorexic is extremely interested in food. This is often expressed through ritualistic and obsessive behaviour:

> I know exactly what I eat each day. It must be exactly the same, I never have anything different. I only eat tinned food, so I know precisely how many calories I've had. If I ever eat fresh food I'd have to weigh it all, and that gets difficult.

The obsessive quality that only allows certain foods to be eaten is effectively communicated to those around her. Working with an anorexic in her family context can feel like entering a strangely distorted world. It seems as if the whole family revolves around the consideration of precisely what she has eaten, and what she will eat. Great lengths may be gone to to make a particular and acceptable food available – the individual obsession becomes a family obsession. Additionally, there is often an extreme interest in buying, preparing, and serving food for others to eat: an anorexic's obsession with food may not allow her to eat for herself, but providing the forbidden fruits for others is pleasurable.

Dunbar's account of Catherine illustrates both this fascination with food and its ability to take others over:

> She would prepare enormous meals for the family and insist that they ate everything, never sitting with us herself. Her tastes in food were bizarre and should anyone walk into a room while she was eating she would either panic and scream or she would become secretive and pretend she wasn't eating. I now see there was a frenzy about her whenever she came into contact with food.[7]

Dunbar later describes how Catherine

> would insist on going inside numerous cafés and looking at the selection of cakes and pastries. By her second day she decided a pastry was what she *had* to have for lunch. If she didn't see *exactly* what she wanted the hunt would be continued, sometimes for two hours.[8]

For those who have not lived with an anorexic, or worked in a family context with one, this anxiety to provide food that is acceptable, and the lengths that will be taken to achieve this, may seem quite incredible. However, the powerful effect on the family reflects something of the girl or woman's experience of anorexia.

Eating disorders and family interactions

It has been argued by some that difficulties in eating arise from particular patterns of interaction in families. Food becomes an interactional commodity – a means of expressing emotions, of conveying messages and making statements. It is a strange, but not altogether ineffective, method of communication, although it begs the obvious question as to what has happened in these families that precludes more direct and straightforward means of interacting.

Since the vast majority of anorexics and bulimics are female, family dynamics may be only one part of the picture, other parts being equally essential. This can only come from awareness of the overall societal context in which women live. Families may be significant, but so is the wider world. Sheila MacLeod reminds us that

> conflicts are partially related to, and arising from, the anorexic's individual history and personality structure – that is, they are intrapsychic. But they are also existential, that is, related to being-in-the-world, which for human beings necessarily means being-in-a-body, and, for women, being in a female body.[9]

However, not forgetting this wider world, it is also important to look at the significance and influence of the smaller world of the family. Families are where children, generally, are brought up: their influence should not be underestimated. Many women with eating disorders describe homes in which issues of control were much in evidence, and where there was little room for negotiation or discussion. One anorexic woman, Emma, described it in this way:

> My father made all the rules. My sister and I had to obey. We were very frightened of him. He'd shout at us, or hit us, and that went on right through our teens. He's always treated us like we were very young. You can't talk to him at all, he won't listen. My mother just does what he says, too. She says it's not worth arguing, because he won't ever change, but she won't leave him either.

Later in therapy, Emma revealed that as a young child she had been sexually abused by her father. Circumstances seemed to suggest that her mother had known of this, although this had never been openly acknowledged. Her relationship with her mother was very intense: it appeared not only that her mother could protect neither of them from her father, but also that she needed her daughter to protect herself. Emma was treated very much as a confidante and friend, at an age when she needed to start becoming a separate and private individual with a life of her own. She experienced her mother as invasive, and her father as abusive and repressive. In this family, with its hidden secret of sexual abuse, there was no room for confrontation, resolution or separation. Emma's entry into, and persistence with, anorexia served many purposes, and it was only through exploring all these that food became less dominant in her life.

Emma's anorexia may help provide some insight into the experiences of other women. First and foremost, food was something she could say 'no' to – successfully. She could not be forced to eat, and, if she did capitulate to pressure, she could induce vomiting and get rid of it all. She could say 'no' to food when she had been unable to say it to her father or to her mother. Her father had invaded her body in particular, and her life more generally, in a way that she had experienced as a violation of her whole self. Her mother, she felt, had colluded, and had, in a different way, also invaded her: she could not let her go to be herself. By the time she was a young adult Emma's sense of self had been sadly eroded. In many senses she was not ready for adulthood, having had so little childhood. This latter point takes us on to the second theme. She was so thin she did not look a woman. She still had the physique of a much younger girl, and the lifestyle to match. She did not have adult relationships. She did not move away from home. Outward signs of her female sexuality were hardly in evidence. She could, in some ways, remain a child in the hope that she might be allowed the childhood previously denied her.

A third theme applied more specifically to her relationship with her mother. Emma felt both rage towards her and tremendous concern for her. Not eating was a way of both expressing this rage and ensuring that she remained living at home, so that she could go on protecting her mother. She felt her mother simply would not be safe without her. This, inevitably, also increased her rage with both parents, but, as with everything else within this family, there was no way of expressing this directly. An indirect expression was the further tightening of the knot of anorexia.

The circularity is obvious: the more pronounced the symptom, the more it becomes the focus of attention within the family. Here, the fourth theme emerged: the symptom was often safer than the underlying causes and became solidly entrenched. It became a dustbin for the ills of the family; everything could be thrown in and the lid firmly closed. Sorting out the mess would have been an unpleasant business, and one that the family members were reluctant to pursue. A neatly defined ill daughter was much more acceptable. Emma would go along with this because she had good reason to believe that if she voiced her underlying concerns, they would be denied, or ignored, thereby increasing her sense of powerlessness.

None of this takes us near the fears and feelings of disintegration that lie hidden within the anorexic. As long as food is experienced as the one aspect of the self that can be contained, controlled and managed, then real desperation, very deep conflicts and unexpressed needs can also be held firmly in check. Refusing food becomes equated with keeping dangerous parts of the self at bay:

> Food, which is usually associated in a person's mind as a positive force has to be, instead, perceived as as negative one. The anorexic woman has transformed the meaning of food in her life so that it becomes designated as dangerous to her well being and survival.[10]

Emma was once asked how it would feel just to be able to allow herself to eat what she would like, with the usual rigid controls removed. Her first response was to feel afraid of even allowing herself to consider the question. She could then see that this was how she would feel about relaxing with food. Even the question and the thought provoked fear; the reality, at that stage, was inconceivable. She felt that if she let go of her control over food, she would be completely lost and quite overwhelmed. It was almost as if her entire self would disappear. Those who knew her at the time were fearful that she might disappear by dying. There was concern that her weight was so low that her life could be threatened. Emma's worry that she could not cope with eating was matched by the contrary concern of others that she would not survive without. Her extreme anxiety and terror when asked about eating, early on in therapy, is well illustrated in her reply:

> Oh, I couldn't, I couldn't, just let myself eat. I don't know what would happen to me. Everything will be all right as long as I stay thin. I can't bear to put on weight. I must know what I'm eating. It's all I think about. It's there all the time. I can't imagine it any different.

Her desperation is hard to convey in print, but the tenaciousness of her position, referred to in Susie Orbach's words above, comes through. Eating disorders really do indicate that a battle is going on inside the person that is not, and cannot, be explicitly expressed. As we have seen with Emma, if the family pattern is one that precludes direct expression, any change is difficult.

Many writers have explored the interactions in such families. Palazzoli[11] sees families with an anorexic as being tightly knit, hard-working and respectable, while also being highly resistant to change or to allowing any individual member expression of his/her individuality. Salvador Minuchin[12] describes these families as enmeshed and rigid – unable to resolve conflict, yet with considerable conflict beneath the surface presentation. For adolescents in these families there is a lack of privacy at an age when they need it. Parents tend to see themselves as having a right to know what others are thinking, and feeling. Hilda Bruch, in her classic study, draws attention to the significance of the anorexic girl's primary relationship with her mother, and also sees the family as creating for her, and in her, a feeling of passivity and powerlessness. Things happen to her; she is not an active agent, but a passive recipient.

Clinical experience suggests that the family of an anorexic or bulimic is frequently one in which a confusing mixture of passivity, anger, distance and apparent closeness exists. The apparent closeness I refer to here is perhaps the 'enmeshment' referred to by Minuchin. The anorexic or bulimic girl or woman will often describe herself as coming from a very close family, or being particularly attached to her mother. As time proceeds, and as trust grows, the picture changes to one in which it seems that the closeness is better described as the desperate bid of a drowning person to clutch at a straw. She simply dare not let go. This may be a bid to protect herself, or other members of the family, or both. She may not be able to let go of them; equally, she is fulfilling an important role within the family, and they may not be able to let go of her.

Secrets are common. In Emma's family the secret was sexual abuse. But there were others, not necessarily so major, but undoubtedly significant, indicating an overall difficulty with communicating. A common pattern within the family is that the mother is the passive partner in the marriage, and the father is both more distant and generally more powerful. Although less likely, it can work the other way around; it seems that it is the imbalance that is important. In such a family, it is unlikely that the growing girl receives either a satisfactory loving relationship or an encouraging model of what adult womanhood can be like. Her sense of her own validity, and of her own rights, is severely limited. There is little awareness of the needs of the growing child, adolescent and young woman. Essentially, she has to fit around the needs of other people. Her voice is not heard, even if she is allowed to use it. Parental needs are paramount, and in a world where power and control are male-dominated, she finds that even in her smaller and more immediate environment she has little say in her own destiny. By definition, she is unable to say that either, since again she will not be heard. In this situation she feels as if her options are severely limited. No wonder that one symptom that achieves so much, in a situation where so few options are available, is held on to so firmly.

Working with women with eating disorders: the process of therapy and counselling

Avoiding participation in the power game

So often the process of working in this area becomes a battle-ground, in which the victor is the one who is able to control the woman's eating, and thereby her body, though not necessarily her independent spirit. Those working in psychiatric hospitals where rituals of observed eating, regular weighing, and systems of rewards are operated, will be familiar with the rules of combat. They will also know that working within this system, it is extremely difficult, particulary for junior members of staff, to query or challenge the regime effectively. While some institutions and agencies give their personnel little choice as to their mode and philosophy of work, some are more flexibile and others are open to challenge. Anorexics who are admitted to hospital can be in a very weak and emaciated state, and death is a very real possibility for some of them. Anxiety about this, and concern about lifesaving, are genuine and need to be seen as such. However, it is still relevant to ask whether or not such methods of treatment really are effective. Perhaps what they do is to intensify the battle for control without acknowledging either the underlying dynamics, or the issues that surround women in relation to food, body size and shape.

Women who have been treated in this way in psychiatric hospitals describe their experience variously:

> Whatever happened to psychotherapy? How can experienced people in the medical profession be so dense as to believe someone with an embedded fear of putting on weight will be cured by a food drip?

> I have suffered from anorexia nervosa for over seven years. I have had hospital treatment for it seven times, which were all very unsuccessful. In fact I would have to say that each period of treatment made my condition worse.

> I was driven into conformity outwardly, but have never been able to really cope. I was horrified by the emphasis placed on feeding anorexic people, to the detriment of any attention paid to the real pains of which the eating problem was a symbol. Nobody cared or even bothered to get to know what I felt like inside. It seemed strange to me that people can be totally oblivious to extreme distress of another. Friendship is a risky thing that most people don't venture into. But it was difficult to take, and confusing from those who profess to care.

This reference to friendship is an interesting one. Other anorexics have mentioned the lack of friendliness towards them when hospitalized. They experienced their treatment as punitive. They felt they were being seen as difficult patients and that they really were embattled. Talking to people who work with eating disorders, this perception does not appear inaccurate. Carers in various professions frequently describe anorexics and bulimics as 'difficult', 'manipulative', 'deceitful' and 'dishonest'. Such value judgements not only effectively obscure the individual from sight, but also firmly and immediately identify the carer as the adversary, who has decided both that there are sides and which side they are on. It is worth noting that attaching these derogatory labels precludes making real contact with the individual. The isolation, hopelessness and anger they already feel is further intensified by dismissive or combative responses.

Other sufferers give a different picture of their treatment under medical and psychiatric care:

> I have endured several types of care, from massive doses of tranquillizers and food on a general medical ward (with no explanation) to long-term psychiatric support. I can now say I am grateful to those people who refused to collude with my illness even when I was desperate for them to do so. I became defensive and secretive in the extreme and unable to see that any alternative to the starvation habit was possible or desirable.

In retrospect, this young woman was grateful for interventions she considered life-saving. But questions remain. Treatment without explanation or real consent, that has to be 'endured', have worrying implications. It seems particularly important when working with the anorexic or bulimic that a real attempt is made to communicate effectively. Otherwise, all too frequently, the pattern of interaction so evident in her family background will simply be repeated. Explanations are not given; discussion is not permitted. Power and control over her own body and self are once again denied her. This is not to say that a co-operative and smooth process can easily be ensured. A rough ride is to be expected. But if the helper does not set out as if entering a battle that has to be won, there is more possibility that ambivalence can be identified and worked with. For those who work in a counselling or therapy mode, it will be evident that at certain points these clients will want to do battle with them. This must be faced and understood. It is, however, very different from deciding at an early stage to enter the battle uninvited, knowing you are on the opposing side. It is far more appropriate to be present as a helpful companion than as a ready-made adversary.

Taking the fear from food

The tension that can surround food and eating has already been referred to. By the time some women come for help, this has reached crisis point. One client describes this:

> Mealtimes are hell. I know what I will eat, and what I won't eat. I cannot eat in front of anyone else. My dad used to insist I eat with the family, but my mum has told him to leave me alone. I eat all by myself, and no one else must see me. No one dares mention food to me now, it's silly really because everyone is just pretending.

The atmosphere in that house at mealtimes can be imagined. It is important that therapy does not become another place where food becomes unmentionable, and where pretence is the name of the game. There is inevitably an uneasy balance between attempting to normalize the subject of food, by discussing it easily and openly and not becoming so obsessed with it that it becomes impossible to look beyond it to the meaning it holds for the client.

There is a danger that each session can be turned into a playback hour, in which every piece of food consumed during the week is reported back. Similarly, it is easy to enter debates, of a semi-intellectual nature, as to the various theories relating to eating disorders. While these may be interesting, they generally do not tend to be helpful, and the therapist or counsellor may need to ask herself/himself what is being avoided at these times. Readers who are not therapists or counsellors may think that those working in this field would not fall into this trap of exchanging information knowledgeably. But they do. Retreating to the firm ground of facts and techniques, even when they are not accurate, can be reassuring to a practitioner, and safe to the client. Particularly with eating disorders, there is again the danger of repeating the family pattern, and of a counsellor or therapist being seen as the parent with special knowledge who must be obeyed.

As with so many other situations, the person who has been approached for help must take care to provide an appropriate balance in his/her work with the client. Changing the subject when food is mentioned, or showing unease oneself, is obviously not encouraging to the client. When food is such a fraught subject, and has so much projected upon it, the helper needs to be able to look at this with the client in a genuinely relaxed manner.

Making sense of the message

Many women who come for help have lived with their eating disorder for many years. It has become part of them, and a part of their way of life. It is familiar, and will often be clung to as if it were a small child's security blanket. It provides an identity and a sense of safety. Considerable fear and anxiety can be engendered at the mere possibility of changing a secure behaviour pattern. Change means that another self will be revealed, and the difficulties and conflicts previously disguised by the obsession with food will become uncovered. By working to understand what has previously been indirectly communicated via eating, it becomes possible to begin to explore the underlying issues. It is not easy to give up a tried and tested security blanket: to take a leap into the unknown can seem dangerous. A vivid description of the difficulty of making such a move is described by a long-term anorexic:

> I have lived with this invisible friend for so long now. I say 'friend' because as time passes, and other things change, anorexia remains faithful, like a favourite pet animal that is always with you. So the hardest part is not admitting or facing your illness honestly, but having the courage to move on into unknown territory.

And for some, that unknown is life as an adult woman:

> I had no desire to grow up. If I didn't grow up, my dad would still love me. I didn't want to lose him. He hated it when my body started to change; he only liked me little. It's still [twenty years later] the one thing I can control, everything else controls me, but no one can make me eat.

Another explains how important weight loss was to her:

> Losing weight is all an anorexic feels she is successful at, so to force her to put on weight is to take away her only lifeline.

Trying to understand the meaning of anorexia and bulimia requires engagement in a real dialogue. When a woman's eating patterns are firmly entrenched, she has often lost contact with the feelings and experiences that triggered this particular response. Tracking this down with her, and starting to explore other avenues, will be frightening. Progress will be erratic, and moves forward will be matched by jumps back into the safety of old patterns that provide comfort. One client commented excitedly:

> Guess what? I was heading straight for the kitchen. I wasn't thinking or feeling, just how I get before I binge, just numb and

empty. And then I stopped and thought about what we had said last week. And I realized I was feeling so angry, that I felt quite murderous. I didn't binge, and I didn't murder anyone, even if part of me would have liked to. I just stormed round for ages feeling furious. I slammed doors and chucked things around – just what I could never do at home. My mum would have had a bad turn, and everything would be my fault.

Being able to link repressed angry feelings with a desire to binge was a crucial step for her, and was an important step in enabling her to effect real changes in her life.

Setting target weights

In short, *don't*. It is too much like entering the client for a competition, with congratulations and praise as the prize. The client may want to please by giving a gift of eating, or may, when angry, wish either to thwart or to worry the counsellor. Either way, setting targets avoids and distorts consideration of the underlying issues.

Women can and do die as a result of anorexia; and very low weight, or eating habits that could be fatal, can be enormously anxiety-provoking. But trying to deal with the anxiety, and attempting to be protective towards the client, cannot be achieved by means that are inherently ineffective. However, it can be useful to attempt to reach an agreement with the client that she will not lose more weight – this is often acceptable to the client, and lessens the therapist's anxieties. It can also be a useful model for the ongoing work – that is, of co-operation with one another. Allowing the anorexic or bulimic client control over her own weight is an essential feature of working with such women. Susie Orbach states that:

> Recovery does not rest on the reversing of the food refusal and restoring weight loss . . . By allowing the processes of learning to eat again and put on weight to remain firmly within the province of the client, the therapeutic partnership can begin the task of understanding the meaning of the food refusal for the individual woman.[13]

It may be difficult for some helpers or the client's family to accept a situation where the client is allowed control over her food intake. It needs to be remembered that forcing food and weight gain are superficial strategies, that have no long-term effectiveness, and are, in any case, open to question in terms of the methods used.

Creating and using the working relationship

Making it clear at an early stage that the client herself has control over her eating, and that the therapist will not make a take-over bid for her body, greatly assists the working relationship. Ensuring that it is understood that food can be discussed without pressure to eat more and differently, can feel very different from previous experiences. It can also help to share with the client an appreciation that her use of food is a way of communicating what is otherwise uncommunicable; and that understanding the complexities of this is not something that will be forced on her, but eventually needs to be examined together.

The relationship needs, essentially, to be a partnership, in which the woman feels safe enough, and accepted enough, to start exploring her own inner anguish. Often the client will experience difficulties and ambivalences in the therapeutic relationship, which will be reflected in other relationships. Frequently, an enormous longing for a close relationship will be matched by fear and mistrust. Sometimes a client will have flitted from one therapist to another. Relationships with people can be deeply confused and confusing. There can be a mixture of great and unexpressed neediness, fear that expression of need will be rejected or overwhelming, and anger that needs will never be met. Within the therapeutic relationship, these issues can begin to be addressed. The client needs to discover that the therapist will not be consumed or overwhelmed by her needs, anger or sadness.

It can be difficult to accept the proffered relationship in therapy. It can be both desired and feared, both accepted and rejected. The counsellor or therapist may well end up feeling, as I explained above, like the food that is so desperately wanted, but denied; like one who occupies so much of the client's time and thoughts, but who is not allowed by her to nourish her. It will take time and tenacity for the relationship to become truly nourishing, one where what is offered can be absorbed calmly, without any desire to spit it out (as food so often can be). Issues of power, control, of meeting and making demands, and of enjoying a closeness which is not open to invasiveness, are equally present in the way food and body image, and being a woman, are pushed upon women in our society, in families and in some forms of treatment. Therapy and counselling require an approach which recognizes all these issues, shares them with the client, and invites her, perhaps for the first time, to confront them for herself.

Notes

1   Winnicott, D.W. (1971). *Playing and Reality*. Tavistock.
2   Garfinkel, P.E. 'The heterogeneity of anorexia nervosa-bulimia as a distinct subgroup', *Archives of General Psychiatry*, 37.
3   Dana, M. and Lawrence, M. (1988). *Women's Secret Disorder: New Understanding of Anorexia*. Grafton Books, p. 26.
4   Orbach, S. (1986). *Hunger Strike*. Faber and Faber, p. 29.
5   Auden, W.H. (1970). *A Certain World*. Faber and Faber.
6   Bruch, H. (1974). *Eating Disorders: Obesity, Anorexia Nervosa, and the Person Within*. Routledge and Kegan Paul.
7   Dunbar, M. (1986). *Catherine: The Story of a Young Girl Who Died of Anorexia*. Viking, p. 34.
8   Ibid., p. 60.
9   MacLeod, S. (1981). *The Art of Starvation*. Virago, p. 11.
10 Orbach, S. *Hunger Strike*, p. 99.
11 Palazzoli, M.S. (1974). *Self Starvation. From the Intrapsychic to the Transpersonal Approach to Anorexia Nervosa*. Human Context Books.
12 Minuchin, S. (1978). *Psychosomatic Families; Anorexia in Context*. Harvard University Press.
13 Orbach, S. *Hunger Strike*, p. 141.

8

Violence against women

I wonder what abuse a woman has to go through at the hands
of a man before she gives up the inward flutter of delight, like
the click and flame of a cheap cigarette lighter, at being
chosen? Where did we learn that definition of honour? As long
as it is there we are never really independent.

Mary Gordon

Women who have experienced violence as a child or as an adult see
the world through different eyes than those who have not. They
frequently express feelings of being alienated, out of step with
others, and of psychological distance. Violence, especially from
those who are apparently to be trusted, is a deep and terrible
assault on the self. Being abused as a child erodes the cornerstone
of the person, and replacing and rebuilding it in adulthood, while
not impossible, is never an easy process. For some women,
violence is an ongoing part of life: abuse at home, bullying at
school, battering from partners. Others, abused as children, may
not enter violent relationships in adulthood. Nevertheless, they
carry within them the experience of earlier assaults, which
inevitably affects their later relationships.

Violence is not confined to individual acts, and is not a modern
syndrome. It can be an approved societal or political response, as is
seen in wartime. The extent of permissible violence depends in
part upon whose side you are on, and the question of whether the
means justify the end assumes paramount importance. Aggression
on a major scale may seem a long way from a child being tortured,
or a wife being battered, but we need to remember that such acts
take place in the context of a world in which torture of children
and adults is commonplace, and often conveniently forgotten.
South and Central America, South Africa and Beirut are sufficiently far away to be dismissed by most of us, most of
the time. Horror rapidly becomes history, but it cannot be
forgotten; nor should we forget that the perpetrators of war, with
a few exceptions, are men, and that those who fight are generally

men. Throughout history men have been reared to enter battle, to fight, and to kill.

Similarly, most violent crimes are committed by men, and this is particularly true of domestic violence. Figures from the Home Office show that in 1986 in England and Wales 60,000 men were cautioned for or prosecuted and found guilty of violent offences, while the number for women was under 6,000. Figures from the United States show that 95 per cent of assaults on spouses and ex-spouses during 1973–7 were committed by men.[1] Historically, men have had considerable rights over their wives – over their property, person, and daily life. Dobash and Dobash[2] suggest that the use of violence in this context has been viewed as a male right, exercised for purposes of control, punishment and domination.

Similarly, violence against children has a long history. The carefully packaged image of the happy nuclear family, lovingly nurturing its children, to which the advertising world adheres so tenaciously, lacks substance beneath the glossy images. Historically, depending on the social class of the family, children have been a source of extra labour or bargaining counters in making advantageous marriages. Children may well have been loved, but they and their mothers were seen as no more than men's possessions. The treatment of children was often brutal. It was not until the late nineteenth century that social reformers became concerned over their condition.

The poor physical state of recruits in the First World War help to heighten awareness. Combined with the publication of, and growing interest in, the work of Freud (in which the significance of early experiences was recognized), there was increasing acknowledgement of childhood as a state and stage of its own. Even so, it was not until the 1940s and 1950s in the United States[3] that doctors began to suspect that some injuries to children were not caused by accident or disease. In 1962 Dr Henry Kempe[4] coined the term 'the battered child syndrome', and this generated an enormous amount of interest and research thereafter.

Those working with women in any context (counselling, social work, the voluntary sector, nursing or psychology) will be familiar with the difficulties for women resulting from exposure to violence. Violence against women is not a rare event; it is horribly common. It frequently takes place within the home, and is frequently not reported to the police. Rape and sexual abuse are often committed by someone known and trusted, and, similarly, often remain a secret. Women who have been abused as children may be many years into their adulthood before they are able to reveal this, despite carrying the heavy burden of such an experience. Working with abused women can uncover an appalling catalogue of brutality, and it is perhaps understandable, although not excusable, that violence has been dismissed as fantasy in some quarters. As with the abuse of children, the reality is so un-acceptable that the appeal of fantasy is considerable.

Working with women abused as children

Child abuse and gender

It should be said that boys as well as girls suffer abuse – sexual or otherwise – in childhood. Given that men commit the majority of violent offences, it is highly probable that more men than women abuse children, and clinical experience further supports this. Research suggests that girls are far more likely to be sexually abused by their fathers or other men, than boys by their mothers or other women. The American Humane Association[5] indicates that with incest, as with other forms of sexual abuse of children, 97 per cent of offenders are male, and 92 per cent of victims are female. Even if this figure is an underestimate of mother–son incest, the evidence certainly suggests that father–daughter incest is a far more extensive problem.

This is not to say that women do not physically and sexually abuse their children, as it is evident that they can and do. However, it is important in understanding the effects on women in later life to recognize the patterns of sexual differentiation that exist. The question of how abuse in childhood may effect men and women differently in adulthood is both complex and important, and needs to be considered in more detail than I have opportunity to do in this book.

To understand how abused women react, the context of their childhood abuse must be recognized. In a patriarchal society, in which, as we have seen, men are well established in positions of power, such blatant misuse of their position from early life on-wards has long-lasting influence on girls and women. Their lack of power becomes double-banked, coming from two sources: patri-archy and male violence.

The powerlessness of the child

Women who have been abused may present as such, but they may come with a variety of other symptoms. Some will never have talked about the experience before. Some will have repressed either the whole experience or certain aspects of it from conscious memory. Uncovering the experience also uncovers fears, anxieties, neediness, insecurities, hurt and rage. When counsellors and therapists work with women who have survived abuse, they are also working with very hurt little girls, betrayed by those they thought they could trust, unable to control what was happening to them. In so many ways they had no power, but, potentially, had so much invested in them. A woman who had been sexually abused by her father recalls being told:

> This is our secret. If you tell, I'll go into a prison and you'll be put in a home. It'll make your Mum ill, and then there'll be no one to look after your brother and sister.

She was powerless to resist her father, while holding, in her young eyes, the potential to destroy the family. If the family split up, it would be her fault. As an adult, giving the responsibility back to her father and disowning it herself was an arduous process. Guilt and responsibility were instilled into her from an early age. Another, physically abused by her father and brother, and bullied at school, describes her response to her treatment:

> I never knew what would happen. Neither of them would ever defend me against the other, and they always used to tell me that it was my fault, that I deserved it. They told me I was bad. My father told me that if I told anyone they'd know I was bad, and I'd get locked up.

The death of trust

It is hardly surprising that, as a young adult, telling or trusting anyone was a huge barrier for this woman to overcome. She feared that she would not be believed, that she or the counsellor would not survive the revelations, that somehow damage would result. As a child she felt overwhelmed by the abuse; she feared she would not survive. Revealing and reliving the experience carried the same fear: she might disintegrate herself, or cause (and perhaps desire) others to do so. In the same way as the early experiences were too much for her as a child, so she feared they would be too much for her counsellor.

This was further complicated by a desire (at least in part) for this to happen – the angry child that wanted the satisfaction of revenge on a brutal and uncomprehending adult world. The untrusting child wanted her view of the world reinforced: that no one would understand, and that nothing would be different. Her despair would remain. Anger would have been expressed but not dealt with. Hope would be quashed and the situation would become more deeply entrenched. However, another part of her, desperately clung on to hope, and to the possibility of change. Her relationship with her counsellor reflected this extreme ambivalence: she would alternate between clinging to the relationship with an intense desire, and pushing it away in extreme fear and anger. Her response when her counsellor was ill, and had to miss a session, typifies this:

> I thought, 'She's just like all the others, I can't trust her'. I didn't want to ever come back, and I didn't care. Later, I just felt so scared in case something had happened to you. I need you to be there, and that makes me want to run away.

Hoping for love

Both the women quoted above had lost much of their childhood. Starting to comprehend the extent of such a huge loss and grieving over this, was a painful process. They had both been abused by male relatives, and had not been protected by their mothers. They were both still in close contact with their families of origin: neither had been given the self-confidence to fully enter the adult world, and it was as if they were still somehow waiting with false hope to receive what they needed but had never received. One of them painfully and vividly expressed this feeling when she told me that she felt like a lost lamb trying to suckle from a dead mother. The image was powerful and evocative: trying in vain for what she knew she would never have, but not quite being able to give up the attempt.

Partners and children

Neither of these women had their own children, and both had difficulties in relating both to men and to women. The one who had been sexually abused struggled against continuing a very destructive pattern of relationships with men. She vacillated between being firmly in control of very unassertive men, and relationships where she was being controlled by an aggressive man. Both were highly unsatisfactory for her, but reflected her confusion and fear of relating. She felt as if she had to be either firmly in control or aggressively controlled. She had no experience of safety in a relationship, of sharing, of compromise, or of care. In her experience being needy or vulnerable led to the worst sort of exploitation. In essence, you had the choice of being the exploited or the exploiter.

The fear both women expressed about the possibility of ever having children came from anxiety that abuse is repeated in families, reinforced by media reporting on abuse. As therapy progressed, this changed for one of them: she realized she could not have prevented her own abuse, but that she did have sufficient power and control over her destiny not to repeat the pattern in her life or in the lives of any children she might have. However, this is a real fear for many women who have survived abuse, creating another potential loss for them: their fear impeding their freedom to choose whether or not to have a child. What has been described here will be a familiar picture both to those who work with abuse survivors and to women who have been abused. It is only a glimpse of what for some is a lifetime's fear and secrecy, a constant experience of a hurt and damaged self that seems impossible to express, and so continually invades present life. It is like living with a ghost which is unseen by others, but is always present, casting a shadow over many aspects of daily life.

Working with women survivors of abuse: the process of therapy and counselling

Disclosure: enabling without pressure

Many abused clients come to see a counsellor or therapist still unable to tell themselves what has happened, let alone anyone else. In my view it is of central importance that the client is not pressurized into revealing details before she is ready. She could not say 'no' to her abuser; she must be able to say 'no' to her counsellor. If she does not feel she can proceed at her own pace, and control what she reveals, she may experience a repetition of earlier abuse. This is a fine balance for the counsellor: on the one hand, she wants to be receptive and facilitative, to hear and acknowledge what is being said; on the other, she must not be invasive.

There is a danger of falling into one of two traps: either becoming another adult who ignores, and does not see or hear; or becoming the person who insensitively takes over without permission. Children who have been abused have frequently been told that they must not tell, and warned of dire consequences if they do. Therapy or counselling gives another message; it is all right to tell and it is safe to do so. However, it may be some time before this message can be believed: a lengthy process of testing may be necessary. Women who were abused as children do not trust easily, so the genuineness of the counsellor's message can only be proved with time.

Boundaries

For a child who suffers abuse, the usual boundaries that exist in a relationship are invaded and demolished. This has implications for the therapeutic relationship. It is important to be clear about the boundaries in counselling. It may reassure the client, and make her feel safer, if boundaries of time, place and length of counselling are clarified. It is important to be reliable and consistent. The client may not be: she may need to miss appointments. She may be late. She may also need to know that her counsellor will stand firm throughout, will not be damaged or upset, and will not take away from her what has been offered.

This is not to say that the counsellor should turn into a passive recipient when boundaries are challenged by the client. Such reactions can be discussed, and the reasons for them understood. This is very different from an authoritarian approach; boundaries exist to provide a safe but gentle holding. They should not become a strangulation. Women who survive abuse can feel tossed around in a sea of pain, uncertainty, and grief. It helps them if the therapist is reasonably securely anchored, and when they know that they themselves will not easily rock the boat.

The hurt child

The woman who has survived abuse as a child carries with her a very hurt small person inside. The counsellor can sometimes feel that she has the child in her counselling room, not the adult. That child must be listened to, and must be heard. She needs to protest, and she needs to grieve. However, the adult in the client has to return to the world after the session. The counsellor's anxiety about this, and perhaps her difficulty in tolerating the intensity of her client's pain, prevent some counsellors from seeing this child. She will not go away if she is not heard, although she may well become repressed, or demonstrate her presence in other ways, particularly through self-harm. This child will have a very poor self-image, which is shared by the adult woman. Either her abuse has been denied, or she has been told that it was her fault and that it was she who was bad.

Counsellors generally prefer to adopt what they see as a neutral, non-judgemental approach to their work. Feminist therapists in some respects diverge from such a stance, and I would argue against neutrality in respect of abuse work. Abuse against children is an adult responsibility; it is never the child's, and it must not be projected on to them. Women survivors have a right to that knowledge, especially where it has hitherto been withheld from them. Counsellors can spell out the innocence of the child to those who have had this taken away from them. Acting as an advocate for the hurt inner child is becoming a more widely accepted model for working with abuse survivors, and the work of Alice Miller has been influential in this respect. She says:

> I always regard myself as the advocate of the child in my patients; whatever they may tell me, I take their side completely, and identify fully with the child in them, who usually is not able to experience his feelings and delegates them to me.[6]

This approach is a long way from the traditionally distant and neutral stance of the analytic therapist, encompassing as it does a belief in firmly taking the side of the hurt child.

Loss, anger, and grieving

Abuse survivors have lost much. Their childhood cannot be recovered, and accepting that is a major ordeal. There can be stages of disbelief, of great distress, and acknowledgement of the loss can lead to enormous anger. This is sometimes expressed in extreme rage towards the therapist or counsellor. It is important not only to contain the anger and despair within a session, so that it does not spill out elsewhere, but also to be able to accept it.

Recalling these earlier events can be a time of major crisis in a client's life; it is useful to check out other sources of support she may have. Offering extra sessions may be necessary. The client needs to know that she cannot hurt or damage the counsellor by letting out her anger. However, containing and accepting is not enough. It is also most important to work with her to understand the source of her rage. In becoming the target for the anger, and allowing her feelings about the abuse to be safely expressed and then understood, the counsellor enables her client to reclaim herself.

For some clients, part of the grieving process involves visiting places or houses where the abuse occurred. Others need to confront their abusers. Some do not need to do this literally; they do it inside themselves. While it is helpful to give opportunity to explore these as possibilities, the client needs to trust herself regarding what will be helpful or unhelpful. She needs to be in control of her own actions, and decisions. What is important is feeling in charge of herself, and taking decisions, rather than the particular choices she makes.

Support for the counsellor

Where counsellors carry much work of this nature (and many people in a whole variety of different settings do), it is essential to have sufficient support. Listening to the details of abuse is not easy. It can be unpleasant, distressing and worrying. Trusted and safe supervision, regular and frequent, is a safeguard for both counsellor and client. A counsellor can easily feel like a saturated sponge. It helps to have someone to throw it at who is resilient enough not to fall over. Abuse survivors have often not learned how to be self-protective. It is important for those working in this field to be able to protect themselves. Constant assessment and self-monitoring help in avoiding too heavy a workload. Self-knowledge and self-awareness are also vital, and if this work touches unresolved aspects of the counsellor's being, then at that point in his/her life it may be better not to take it on.

Working with women living with violent partners

Past and present: women and violence

The 1970s saw a renewed awareness of the problem of 'battered wives' with the opening of refuges for women, but domestic violence has a long history: A man's right to beat his wife was firmly entrenched in British law until the late nineteenth century, the only controversial issue until then being what the acceptable limits were to such treatment.[7]

It is paradoxical that for abused women and children, the home is the place of greatest threat. For most of us, it is a safe place to retreat to. Evidence from women's refuges, and from several studies, for example those of Pahl[8] and Bowker,[9] gives a clear indication that the level of violence suffered by women is serious and extensive. Lorna Smith points out that:

> Despite disagreement over many aspects of domestic violence by various researchers, one of the few things about which there is almost universal agreement is that it escalates in frequency and intensity over time. Numerous studies have exploded the myth that serious injuries seldom occur or that weapons are seldom used. If violence happens once, it is likely to happen often.[10]

Women who have been subjected to violence, especially in the early stages of a relationship, can appear convinced that change will occur, and violence will cease, particularly when the attack is followed by contrite apology. The following extract comes from the first counselling session with a young woman who had left her boyfriend after a serious attack on her. In their short relationship, she had already been badly hurt twice:

> Well, of course, he's not really a violent person. I mean, he's terribly upset afterwards, and it's always when he's been drinking. But I know it's dangerous: he did knock me out, and I suppose I'm lucky he didn't kill me. Everybody keeps telling me that once a man starts being violent he won't change. But I can't believe that, can you? I really need a bit of time to think it all over, but he's so sorry he won't leave me alone, he keeps coming round. If I go back to him I think it will be all right. I think he'll know he mustn't do it again, after all he knows I'll walk out.

She did go back; the violence, predictably, occurred again. In this instance, this woman was not restricted, as so many women are, by economic factors, by lack of housing, by dependent children. She was able to support herself financially, and had her own accommodation. Whatever drew her to, and kept her in, a relationship that was life-threatening, appeared to come from within her. On one level she was fortunate: she did have choices. On another, this was evidently not the case. Something prevented the choices from being translated into reality.

Women and separateness: why women don't leave

We have seen in an earlier chapter that women tend to define themselves in terms of their relationships with men, and that when a relationship ends, or goes wrong, they experience a sense of loss of self. We have also seen how women are disadvantaged in the job market, and, therefore, financially; and how difficult it is for women to bring up children single-handedly, although many do so successfully, against the odds. These factors operate together to maintain women in relationships that are violent.

It is very difficult to leave a relationship when doing so makes you feel a failure, when you know you cannot adequately support your children (especially when state support is a passport to poverty), and when abuse has left you demoralized, frightened, and defeated. To leave a partnership under these conditions needs a considerable degree of courage, desperation, assertiveness and self-protectiveness. Violence can induce a feeling of numbness, non-existence and psychological paralysis. Small wonder that leaving is so difficult. .

Men who are violent have real power over women, and they use it. Women know what this has done to them, and they live with fear. Leaving a violent partner does not always remove a woman's fear; she often lives in terror of pursuit and retaliation, accompanied by an anxiety that the law will not afford her adequate protection. Many a woman's previous experience has been that her partner's violence has been unstoppable.

Some women appear to fall into a pattern that could be seen as a false and distorted maternalism towards men. This may not be surprising, as this is a role that is universally acclaimed and approved of for women, and one which does give them some status and limited power. The syndrome can manifest itself in many ways: 'I must get back and cook his tea, he can only just manage to boil an egg, and you should see the mess he makes' is a typical expression of it. Another is: 'Well, he works hard, he needs his relaxation; he always goes to the pub/ goes fishing/ plays golf/ watches football'. The man becomes the child: he cannot be expected to take care of himself, and he must have his playtime. This may be one way of dealing with someone who in so many ways has more power and authority: the idea of 'they're all little boys at heart' perhaps reduces men to a more manageable size. But when extended to indulging, and excusing, violent behaviour the distortion becomes potentially life-threatening. Consider the following words from a wife following another attack by her husband:

I can just be sitting there and he'll be walking through the door and he'll just throw me on the ground and start kicking me. I think he thinks it's his right really – his dad is like that with his mum. But he's really very fond of me and he's often ever so sorry afterwards and ever so nice. And I suppose I'm not a very good wife to him, my job is important to me, and he doesn't like it when I'm back late and he's waiting for his tea. I think it might be up to me, you know, to avoid situations when he might be violent. After all, he can't really help it – I mean they can't, can they? It all just gets too much and he explodes, poor thing.

It is not a truculent and tired three-year-old in a tantrum who is being described here, but a grown man whose violence has already once led to his wife's hospitalization.

Repeating patterns

Popularly held opinion maintains the idea of the cycle of violence: that men and women abused as children somehow seek one another out in adulthood and continue the pattern into their own adulthood and, indeed, often into the treatment of their children. In this analysis pain and pleasure, love and torture, become inextricably linked. Erin Pizzey and Jeff Shapiro[11] have described how they believe this explains the behaviour of both abused and abuser, and the tenacity of such couples in clinging to abuse. If they manage to leave one violent relationship, they will enter another. However, although this may apply to some situations, and there is evidence that it does, it is not a universal explanation, and should not be treated as such. As an explanation it is horribly near to the twin myths of 'women ask for it', and 'they enjoy it'. Such myths can all too easily prevent serious attention from being paid to domestic violence. Explanations that look only at individual pathology, and ignore the wider picture, need to be viewed with caution. It is easy to regard abused women as disturbed, neurotic or mentally ill without realizing that it is violence that can make them so.

The other side of this argument is illustrated by the findings of a study carried out by B. Andrews[12]. Out of a sample of fifty-nine women victims of domestic violence, only three entered a new violent relationship, having previously left one. It seems more likely that the behaviour of the abusing man can be explained by a violent childhood. A study by D. Martin and D.S. Kalmuss[13] shows that it is not women victims who come from abusive families; it is male aggressors who do. Many women are able to leave violent relationships, although it is never an easy thing to do. The following words come from a session with a woman with a small child and no independent income, who stayed in temporary accommodation for many months after leaving her partner. Her words illustrate how demoralizing violence can be:

> What you said last time really made sense [that her partner was turning her into a powerless, defenceless child]. He's turned me into a little girl; he's taken away my adulthood. He's got no right to do that to me. He says things like: 'You've been a good girl today' or 'You've been bad; you deserve to be punished' or 'I'm only violent because you deserve it, because you can be so annoying – you answer back' or 'If you were reasonable you wouldn't make me hurt you'. After a while I start to believe he's right, and I think, 'I'm going mad'.

This woman did manage to leave. Doing so produced a real crisis of self-confidence in her, and she lived in abject terror for some time. She was not able to go out alone, and she suffered nightmares for a long period of time. However, she began to rebuild her life successfully, to discover and enjoy herself.

Working with women in violent relationships: the process of therapy and counselling

Unravelling the practical from the psychological

Understanding how women subjected to violence make sense of it, and looking with them at why they stay with violent partners, is of obvious importance. However, some who come into contact with abused women make the assumption, especially where violence has continued over a period of time, that the woman must somehow be colluding with or enjoying it, or that she would otherwise leave. Violent treatment can become a way of life; demoralization and fear can be so all-encompassing that they wipe out any ability to question, think or feel.

Not all women who are abused by partners will present that as their problem. They may be aware of feeling depressed, tired, anxious and hopeless, but will not have connected this with how they are being treated. They see no way out, and feel there is no point in talking about it – it is just the way things are. If violence has been part of a way of life, someone else enquiring about it, and encouraging them to enquire into it, can seem strange. Connecting the violence with, for example, depression, may seem obvious to the counsellor but not to the client.

If a woman says that she would leave, but has no money, no accommodation and no job, or that she believes that her husband would come after her, these are real problems. They should be acknowledged as such. They can be extraordinarily difficult, though not always impossible, to overcome. That needs to be stated. Leaving is not easy; knowing that it is a problematic situation, rather than feeling individually responsible for finding it hard, can be reassuring. It should never be forgotten that fear of retaliation is a powerful reason for not leaving. Women can and do run away, only to be found, brought back and subjected to even worse treatment.

In this situation, it is quite clear that psychological help is inappropriate as an initial or only response. The counsellor may not have the skill or knowledge necessary to assist with these difficulties. But if they are not addressed, and not taken seriously, other forms of intervention will be ineffective. Other agencies may be able to work with the client, as an advocate, to help with these crucial practical difficulties. If she is worn out, depressed and scared, she will need help in seeking the legal, medical, financial and housing assistance that she needs. You have to feel at your best, not your worst, to deal effectively with a complex of agencies and professionals, yet this is not how abused women feel. A woman trying to leave a violent relationship must be given every chance to do so. If she is not met with a prompt and positive response, she can find it even more difficult to request help on future occasions.

Others present themselves as wishing to leave a violent partner, particularly if there has been a recent and serious assault, but then seem unable to do so, even if economically they are able to support themselves and their children. Similarly, when practical support is offered to women who say they would leave if they could, they do not always do so. Other factors are then at work, and if they are not identified and worked with, what is an intolerable situation will simply remain unchanged. This can take a variety of forms.

'I can't manage alone'

A woman who has experienced violence can feel so deflated and devalued that she cannot imagine being able to cope alone. If this is further reinforced by feeling that it is her fault that the marriage has gone wrong – often emphasized by her partner – her self-esteem is in danger of dying completely.

It is important to understand what can be meant by phrases like 'I can't cope alone', and to help the client to understand this. It is likely that she cannot conceive ever feeling different. Furthermore, there is the additional pressure that being alone carries some social unacceptability. There seems no way forward. Resurrecting hope is a struggle. Her right to despair, and for this to be heard, is important. It is not helpful, although it may feel comforting to the counsellor, energetically to rush into consultations with, for example, housing departments, when the client may not yet be ready. If her despair, and anger are not given space for expression, they will sabotage other attempts at help.

This balance has to be reached sensitively: if practical resources are not offered when needed, the client may feel rejected, and withdraw; if they are offered when not appropriate, she will not be able to accept them. The danger is then that when she finally wants help she will have alienated those in a position to offer it, by earlier refusing it. It can be helpful, as a counsellor, to be open about this predicament with the client. The client is often not aware of this problem, but may be able to recognize what is happening when it is discussed. It opens the door to a mutual assessment of what might be most helpful at what stage. Recognizing the possibility of sabotage can make the situation more manageable.

Paradoxically, a woman often fears her ability to be alone, when the reality, as others see it, suggests that her relationship is so destructive that, far from offering any support, it knocks her down emotionally and physically. Essentially, she is already alone, and common sense suggests that she would be better off literally alone. This awareness, often so obvious to both friends and those in the caring professions, can cause them to become irritated and exasperated with her when she does not leave. Ultimately, if their sympathy and support is withdrawn, she is left even more alone and alienated, and finds it still harder to leave. A vicious circle draws tighter. Therapists and counsellors need to be able to recognize the possibility that this cycle exists: acknowledging it gives a chance of escape but denial reinforces it.

It needs to be remembered that a further layer to the anxiously expressed 'I can't manage alone' is provided by a pervasive societal message: that a woman needs a man to care for her. It is not easy for women to live alone. There is no obvious recognizable and acceptable niche for them to slot into. Women who do live alone and enjoy it are often surprised that they do because society is strongly couple-orientated. The discovery that there are alternatives can be unexpected. Many women who are struggling to leave violent relationships have frequently had little or no experience of living and acting independently. The thought of doing so is frightening. Awareness of these issues in working with abused women is essential. If the context is not appreciated, and worked with, it is all too easy to fall into the judgemental responses that are heard, such as 'She won't be helped', 'She could leave if she wanted to' and 'She must like it really'.

Working with ambivalence

It is not easy to leave an established relationship. The existence of violence within it does not magically make it any different, as the following words demonstrate:

> It's the sort of thing we've discussed at women's groups. You know, what you'd do if your partner was ever violent. Well, that's an easy one, isn't it. I'm a feminist; I'm independent; I feel fiercely about women's rights. No man would ever do that to me. The answer clearly was: the relationship would end. I would leave, or he would go. That would be that. But, when it happened, it didn't feel that easy. Something must be wrong; he must be ill – having a breakdown. This couldn't really be happening. He wasn't like that. I wouldn't be with that sort of man. I couldn't have got it that wrong. I didn't understand. I couldn't just leave. I needed to understand what had happened. And for a while it was lovely. I was so glad that it was all right: it really was an isolated incident. But it wasn't. It took me a long while to recognize that. And by then I was so depressed, so stunned, that doing anything was hard, and making a major life decision, with all the practical difficulties that involved, felt impossible. I did it. But the pain, the heartache were dreadful.

The sense of disbelief, shock, questioning, and shattered hopes and dreams, is very evident. The pattern of attack followed by reconciliation and the renewal of hope, only to have it shattered again, is a familiar one. Generally people enter relationships hoping and believing that they will last, trusting that they have chosen the right person, and believing that the person they have chosen is trustworthy. Discovering that it is no longer so is always a shock, and violence is a particularly brutal road to that recognition. The situation can be a very confusing one: in between the bouts of violence there can be loving and happy moments. It is a dilemma: which message to believe? Inevitably, it is preferable for most women to believe the loving message. The situation may seem clear-cut to those outside: violence is not acceptable, therefore it would be best to end the relationship. But it is not always so simple from the inside.

For a woman to leave any relationship can involve mixed feelings, and leaving a violent man especially so. She may well want to leave the violent parts, but not the whole. Really, she wants the situation to change, rather than to give up on it. Perhaps we would all like to feel that we would not tolerate abuse against ourselves, and that we would never be abusive. Perhaps when women are as deeply ambivalent as they can be about leaving a violent relationship, it is deeply threatening to others. Certainly, it seems easy for people to become quite antagonistic towards women who express ambivalence, which makes it hard for them to acknowledge these very confusing feelings. Yet, in order to find a way through, women need to be helped to express and accept that they are confused; that confusion, although unpleasant, is acceptable and, given the situation, appropriate. If they can understand the source of these feelings, they are far more likely to be in control of them and able to start making decisions. It is simplistic and unhelpful to suggest the possibility, or desirability, of anything certain, in a situation that renders clarity difficult and certainty highly unlikely.

Taking back power

The woman who recognized that her husband was treating her as a child, and not as an adult, was able to see that he had effectively knocked away all her adult coping strategies. She was quite clear that she would not tolerate that sort of treatment from anyone else, and indeed had not been treated like that as a child. It felt, talking to her, that in effect she had been brainwashed. The combination of physical violence and ongoing personal denigration, had completely removed, for the time being, her adult coping self in relation to her husband. She was completely powerless. This feeling extended into the rest of her world, although not to such a marked extent.

Helping women to look at how they may recover their power is not an easy task. Challenging a violent man can produce more abuse as he attempts to maintain his power:

> While some women find the violence directed at them to be unanticipated, others report that, as long as the men they live with are not challenged or disobeyed, no abuse occurs or it is limited. As is true of oppressed people generally, women who live with violent men study their behaviour closely in order to be able to avoid violent encounters.[14]

For some women, recovering their adult autonomy and power is a slow process. It starts with the decision to separate, but continues for a long while afterwards. Counsellors can aid this process by offering a safe and reliable relationship and environment. Leaving violence behind does not take the memories or the effects away. The woman will need considerable encouragement and reinforcement, and an opportunity to try to make sense of her life. Having the space to do that can be frightening in itself. A new focus for living has to be found, and other relationships reassessed. When a previously abused woman starts making changes for herself, this can be an enormous delight to her and to her therapist. One woman, in a state of high excitement, reported the following:

> You'll never guess what I did. I told him to leave me alone; never to dare to touch me again. That I didn't care if he was in charge. That he didn't own me. And that if I had any more of that nonsense, I was reporting him to his manager, and I'd go to the union. He sort of crept away and he's been all right since. And I really mean it.

The man in question had been harassing her at work, causing her great distress. When she was able to recognise that he created the same feelings in her that her husband had done, she started reassessing the situation. After much discussion, and carefully looking at her options, and the possible outcome of these, she came to a decision and acted accordingly. This marked a very significant step forward for her. She had been made powerless by her husband. But in some situations she did have power if she was able to exercise it.

It may seem to the reader an obvious link for her to make: that other men could frighten her as her husband had done. In fact, recognizing this was not easy for her, and it took some weeks' work before she was able to appreciate the depth of her fear, the extent of her feelings of powerlessness, and how this had become extended to all her relationships. Ultimately this recognition, combined with identifying and discussing possible strategies, and supporting her right not to be harassed, enabled her to act effectively and assertively.

Working with rape victims

Women in danger

Rape is not an unusual occurrence. The number of reported rapes is nowhere near the actual number of victims. In my own clinical work, only one rape victim reported the attack to the police; I have lost count of the others who reported nothing. Rape is primarily a violent and criminal attack; it should not be classed as a sexual experience. It humiliates, degrades and terrifies, and it is intended to do so. It is the greatest possible invasion of a woman's body and self, against her wishes, and without her consent. She often feels her life is in danger, and, indeed, the use, or threat of use, of knives and other weapons is common.

Women are warned against the dangers of walking alone at night: they should avoid alleyways and unlit roads; they should keep within sight and sound of occupied houses; they should not walk in the shade of trees and bushes; they should be watchful; they should carry alarms; they should avoid direct eye contact. Women have an enormous responsibility placed on them, to protect themselves and to keep themselves safe. It is almost like living under curfew. The threat and fear of attack is huge for women, and is based on reality.

In fact, many rapes are carried out by men known to the victim, sometimes well known, sometimes only slightly. Rape can occur at any time of day or night, and it is not always in a dark alleyway. Rape frequently occurs in a woman's own home; even what was felt to be a safe place becomes tainted and spoilt.

Where is the responsibility of men? Given that attacks on women are mainly carried out by men, and all rapes are by men, what about some controls on them? If anyone should be restricted after dark, perhaps it should be men who are kept inside. Perhaps there should be more emphasis on men taking care; of acknowledging and respecting the rights of women. Perhaps more men should get angry about violence to women. It seems reasonable to pose the question: why are more men not actively protesting? In reality, neither men nor women can be restricted in their movements, although considerable attempts are made to impose such restrictions on women. But the emphasis on women needing to keep safe implies that men are a lost cause. Women have to accept that and to beware. Somehow, that seems most unsatisfactory.

'Women ask for it'

Women are all too easily blamed for rape:

> Both men and women tend to blame the rape victim, although their reasons for placing the blame differ. Men are more likely to assume that the woman unconsciously wanted to be raped and was seductive: her clothes and appearance were too sexy, or she led the rapist on and then changed her mind. Women, on the other hand, tend to blame the woman for simply being in the wrong place at the wrong time.[15]

Blaming women for rape is another means of emphasizing the victim and playing down the role of her attacker. It also assumes, for example, that if a woman is dressed attractively she is issuing an invitation to a man; or that if she is out late at night, that is provocative. Men who dress to accentuate their sexuality, and stay out late, are not perceived in the same way. Women not only have to cope with the appalling trauma of rape, but also are faced, all too often, with a sceptical world that holds them responsible.

Perhaps it is comforting for women to believe that if they are careful, and obey certain rules, they will be protected. A woman who is raped must have broken the rules, and failed to take sufficient care. If she had done she would have been safe. Similarly, men who rape are somehow viewed as a different species. Both men and women can collude in this belief. It moves reality into the realm of the sick and the mad, and away from men and male responsibility.

A man will protect you?

Rape can be a sudden attack by a total stranger, but often it is not. Women are frequently raped by partners. (Although rape within marriage is a contentious issue women certainly experience this.) They can be raped by acquaintances, colleagues, neighbours, former partners and friends. The betrayal of trust in these instances is overwhelming and bewildering. The question 'How could he do that to me?' is one which women painfully ask and cannot answer. Rape, in these circumstances, is rarely reported, and none of the women quoted below would even consider going to the police.

One woman describes her experience:

> I've known him for ages. He'd drink in the bar with his students. I
> went with him to his room to get a book I wanted to borrow. That's
> when it happened. I couldn't believe it was happening. He took no
> notice of me; he wouldn't listen. I didn't realize just how physically
> strong a man can be. Afterwards he said 'I've always wanted to do
> that to a lesbian'. He told me that if I was thinking of telling anyone,
> there was no point. No one would believe me, and he'd say I said
> 'yes'.

The man in question was, in fact, a pillar of the community, well
known in his locality, a professional, married man with children.
She felt she would not be believed, and that the trauma would be
made even worse. A few weeks later she attempted suicide.

Another woman describes her terror:

> I'd broken off the relationship with him, but I'd tried to keep things
> friendly; I had to really, because there were a lot of things that had
> to be sorted out. And, anyway, we'd had good times, and there's no
> need to get nasty, just because it doesn't work. We were going out
> for a meal. We agreed to do that, and sort out some outstanding
> money. On the way there he drove off the main road, and he raped
> me. I did fight and scream. There was no one to hear, and it seemed
> to excite him. I can't describe the terror I felt. I suddenly thought:
> this is how women get killed. I stopped fighting then. I didn't want
> to die.

Her rapist, frighteningly, had a job where he exercised power and
control over the lives of other people, and, even more worrying,
over people who were themselves in a vulnerable state.

Another victim describes staying with her friend in a house
shared by a group of men and women:

> I was woken in the night by one of them, who I knew slightly. He
> got into bed with me, gagged me, and raped me. It was like a
> nightmare. He didn't say anything. I saw him in the morning,
> having breakfast with one of the other women, who is his
> girlfriend. I was numb and terrified. I did tell my friend. She wanted
> me to go to the police, but I couldn't have gone through that as well.

It is often assumed that rape by a person known to the victim is
in some way an 'invited rape' – that somehow signals have been
given, that the woman really wanted the man. This is not the case.
In all these instances, and in many more I could cite, the victim
assumed that she was safe with a man who was known to her and
apparently trustworthy. These men proved not to be so. But

unless these women had led their lives in a constant state of high suspicion and cynicism, their trust was, as far as they could gauge, justified.

Working with rape victims: the process of counselling and therapy

Immediate responses

The implications for the counsellor of working with rape victims depend in part on whether the rape has just occurred, or whether it has been finally acknowledged by the victim years after the event.

If a woman presents soon after the event, then clearly she is in an immediate crisis which demands a particular response. Holmstrom and Burgess[16] suggest that the victim is treated as a customer, and that the counsellor should therefore pay careful attention to her requests, taking these seriously and, as far as possible, meeting them. These crisis requests fall into several categories, including the question of possible police intervention, requests for psychological help, and the need for medical care.

Crisis intervention techniques essentially focus on the crisis of the moment; past experiences and history, are not, at that time, relevant. Meeting the particular needs of rape victims immediately after the attack is important: my own clinical experience is that intervention at an early stage, geared to the individual's expressed needs, enables a more rapid recovery. At this time, the victim is likely to need to make decisions about involving the police, and will require accurate information about the legal process involved. Whatever her decision, it has to be hers, and she will need support for her decision, whatever it may be. She must not be pressurized by anyone – it is crucial that she is able to decide independently.

Younger victims are faced with the dilemma of whether they tell their parents. They may not be able to do this alone, and it can be helpful if their counsellor is present. If this is done, it is important to be quite clear beforehand what the client wishes you to say, and what must remain confidential. Having had no control over what has happened to her, she must be given as much control as possible in the counselling process. Once parents have been told, the victim is often left feeling greatly relieved. But her parents may be very shocked and need help in their own right, to cope with both their daughter's distress and their own.

Recalling the rape

Recalling the detail of the assault, often repeating this over and over again, is helpful and necessary. The victim not only needs to do this at the time of the assault, but often for a long while afterwards. She is likely to need reassurance from her counsellor that she can do just that, in as much detail and for as long as she needs to. It can be difficult for her to do this with friends and family, even those who know what has happened to her. She may feel that they cannot cope, and she may be correct. It is not comfortable to listen to details which are often horrifying. It is hard to be with someone in such psychological agony and distress.

She may worry that no one can bear to be with her when she feels so awful. Such a feeling is apparent in the initial period following a rape. At first she can talk about it but as time goes on she feels it becomes less acceptable. Often her anxiety will be that if she expresses how awful she feels, people around her will not cope with it. One victim expressed it in this way:

> I can't keep going on about it. It's like a nightmare. I can tell nobody wants to hear it again. It's too much for them. They can't handle it. It's hurting them.

When she said this in the session, everything felt completely stuck. She could say nothing, and found it hard even to look at her counsellor. Three things had to be said by the counsellor before any headway could be made. The first was to acknowledge the client's anxiety that her counsellor might not want to hear her talk about the rape, and would not be able to cope. It was very important to reassure her that this was not so. Second, it was necessary to suggest that her fear that no one could tolerate her recounting the experience very much reflected her experience of the rape. It had been so intolerable, and so awful to her, that she had felt, and still felt, that she herself could not cope. The third intervention is central, and deserves a section to itself.

Anger

The third aspect, handled with enormous care, was a guess, but one which was acknowledged as correct. The counsellor attempted to draw out the angry feelings which the client might be experiencing. The counsellor suggested that such a dreadful assault had perhaps left her very angry, as well as extremely distressed and hurt; it might be more difficult to show the anger, especially if she also felt angry with those she needed. The client was able to acknowledge that she was indeed frightened by her desire both to be very angry and to hurt those close to her. Part of her wanted to be intolerable to them, so they would know how bad she felt, and so that in some way she could retaliate for what had happened to her. Another part of her was genuinely protective to those around her.

Her counsellor was able to recognize this protectiveness and at the same time allow the anger to be expressed, knowing that it would not be destructive to either of them. Unexpressed, there was a danger that the client would not have returned for further sessions, or that her feelings could have become translated into actual destructive actions.

Rape can also induce feelings of absolute fury in those who work with the victims, rage which feels entirely appropriate. However, care must be taken that the counsellor's outrage does not overwhelm considerations of what the client needs. In fact, the anger of the counsellor is often in direct contrast to apparent lack of it in the client. Rape victims frequently do not appear to be angry. When they start feeling and expressing anger, it can be the beginning of the process of recovery.

It is important, as illustrated above, to be sensitive to when a woman is feeling anger, and to be able to look at this with her. On the occasion under discussion, the counsellor herself was very aware of her own anger with the unknown rapist. Her caution in responding to her client arose partly from her awareness that this was a sensitive area, partly also because of her uncertainty about projecting her own angry feelings onto her client. This is a useful illustration of a golden rule in therapy and counselling: if in doubt be tentative; certainly be aware of your own feelings, but do not assume that they always reflect your client's experience. They may, but that needs confirmation by the only person who knows – the client. This is particularly true in working with rape victims since rape arouses such powerful feelings.

'I must have deserved it'

The experience of rape is devastating. The lack of expressed anger towards the perpetrator, especially in the early days and months after the attack, is partly explained by the victim feeling that she was herself to blame; and that she must have deserved it. That such a terrible thing should happen, that has made her feel so bad, can only have occurred because she was bad: this may not seem rational, but it is a very real feeling. It is as if she was so powerless to resist what was an appalling act against her, that the badness of the act enters her so deeply, that she herself becomes bad, and cannot resist that either. Rape victims feel dirty; an immediate response after a rape is often to throw away their clothes. Continual bathing can become a way of life, but the feeling does not go away easily. One victim describes her feeling of being bad, and of feeling dirty:

> I can't escape it. I must have deserved it; I must be a really bad person. He wouldn't have done it otherwise, would he? I wish I could stop feeling so dirty. It's unbearable, I just keep trying to wash it all away, and nothing helps.

As with making clear the responsibility of the adult in the abuse of a child so the counsellor can assert the total and absolute responsibility of the perpetrator for rape. This will need ongoing repetition so that the victim can reach a point where she challenges her view of herself as guilty. Recognizing that powerful and violent acts have powerful and violent consequences also assists the victim in reviewing her own negative self-image.

Delayed recognition

Some rape victims supress the experience for a long time. Memories are triggered by a television programme, an article, or friends discussing rape. Whatever the trigger, the effect is considerable. It is much more difficult to tell family and friends long after the event, so support may be limited, and reactions various.

Although the process of working is similar to when the attack is revealed immediately, it needs to be recognized that the shock of revived memory is severe. Counsellors need to be aware of this, and also that support may not be forthcoming from others. Although it is not appropriate in early sessions, it is worth considering the reasons for the repression of so momentous a trauma. It could, for instance, reflect other patterns in her life of major events being ignored, or significant others not being trustworthy. A woman who has been raped more than once can find disclosure particularly threatening. She will fear that others will assume that it must have been her fault.

Moving on

Rape inevitably has serious consequences for the victim's relationships, especially with men. Any sexual activity can become abhorrent, and this can cause great distress in an existing relationship, or can prevent the formation of new ones. Distress is also caused to the partner; he, too, may feel guilty, helpless, angry and powerless, and at a loss to know how best to help. Couple therapy may be appropriate at some stage, or the partner may need a chance to talk in his own right.

Most rape victims wish to be able to resume satisfactory relationships with men. When a client expresses this, it is important to acknowledge it, and to work with her to enable her to achieve what she wishes. In this sense it is not appropriate to adopt an anti-male stance. There is excellent reason unreservedly to uphold a woman's right to not be the victim of attack, but an anti-rape stance should not extend to an implication that all men are bad. Rape victims are vulnerable; dogmatic ideologies must not be imposed upon them.

Violence: an overview

There is nothing like condensing such a massive subject into so few pages to bring home the horrifying extent of violence against women and girls. It would be easy to be overwhelmed by it, to decide to look away, to turn the spotlight on another angle.

But there is hope there, too. Women are impressive in their ability to survive. Many women have appalling stories of abuse to tell. They carry physical and emotional scars. But they fight on and come out winning. Many give excellent care to their children and to others. They value life but never take it for granted. Others do not survive, or do so by the skin of their teeth. Their quality of life is unacceptably low, and the treatment they receive should not be tolerated. Therapists and counsellors, while gaining strength and hope from the one group, should not forget those who are less able, for one reason or another, to come through.

Notes

1   U.S. Department of Justice (1983). Report to the Nation on Crime and Justice: The Data. Washington, DC: Bureau of Justice Statistics.
2   Dobash, R.E. and Dobash, R.P. (1981). 'Community response to

violence against wives: charivari, abstract justice and patriarchy', *Social Problems* 28, 5, pp. 563–81.

3 Woolley, P.V. and Evans, W.A. (1955). 'The significance of skeletal lesions in infants resembling those of traumatic origin', *Journal of the American Medical Association*, 158, 7, pp. 539–43.

4 Kempe, H. (1962). 'The battered child syndrome', *Journal of the American Medical Association*, 181, 17–22.

5 DeFrancis, V. (ed.) (1967). *Sexual Abuse of Children*. Denver, Col.: American Humane Association.

6 Miller, A. (1984). *Thou Shalt Not Be Aware*. Pluto Press, p. 59.

7 Binney, V. (1981). 'Domestic Violence: Battered Women in Britain in the 1970s' in Cambridge Women's Studies Group (eds) *Women in Society*. Virago, p. 115.

8 Pahl, J. (ed.) (1985). *Private Violence and Public Policy*. Routledge and Kegan Paul.

9 Bowker, L. (1983). *Beating Wife Beating*. Lexington, Mass.: Lexington Books.

10 Smith, L. (1989). *Domestic Violence: an overview of the literature*. HMSO, p. 16.

11 Pizzey, E. and Shapiro, J. (1982). *Prone to Violence*. Hamlyn.

12 Andrews, B. (1987). 'Violence in Normal Families'. Paper presented to *Marriage Research Centre Conference on Family Violence*, London.

13 Martin, D. (1976). *Battered Wives*. San Francisco: Glide Publications.

14 Hanma, J. and Saunders, S. (1984). *Well-Founded Fear: a Community Study of Violence to Women*. Hutchinson, p. 87.

15 Rohrbaugh, J.B. (1981). *Women: Psychology's Puzzle*. Sphere Books, p. 291.

16 Holmstrom, L. and Burgess, A. (1974). *Rape: Victims of Crisis*. Bowie, Maryland: Brady.

9

Coming out of the shadows

If the first woman God ever made
was strong enough to turn the world
upside down, all alone,
together women ought to be able to turn it
right side up again.

Erlene Stetson

Any system that gives power to a particular group invites and
encourages the oppression of those who, by reason of gender,
class, race, education, economic or other status, are not eligible for
membership of that group. Patriarchy is no exception to this; in
fact, it is an outstanding example. For although we have come a
long way since the days when women were not allowed to vote,
and were effectively owned, first by their fathers and then by their
husbands, the journey ahead remains a long one. Equal rights may
now be on the agenda, but, as we have seen in earlier chapters,
words have not as yet been fully matched by action. It is
undoubtedly now less easy in Britain to discriminate against
women, but discrimination is still present, albeit less blatant than
formerly. Legislative changes and pressure from women's groups
have resulted in greater awareness of women's rights. However,
male rhetoric on this subject often bears little resemblance to the
reality of how men actually respond to and treat women. So
although progress is being made, changes are apparent, and hope
is on the horizon, there is a long way to go, and it can seem an
uphill struggle.

The importance of understanding the systems and society in
which women live has been stressed throughout this book. If
counselling and therapy are to free them, rather than to freeze
them, in uncovering choices, and to lift them from, rather than
smother them with a blanket of oppression, then they should not
be viewed in isolation. Essentially, they are part of a larger whole
over which they have had little control historically, and which has
severely limited their choices. Additionally, society has systemati-
cally and consistently failed to acknowledge the value of the

contributions women have made throughout history to the maintenance and survival of the whole. The unsung heroes of history are heroines.

In a parallel way, women need to be regarded as individuals, and not just as part of an amorphous mass; each one exists in her own right, and is entitled to make her choices relating to the path her individual life might take. Whether this path leads to a life centred on work and career, or on the home and family, or incorporates both, she needs to know and to feel that she and her way of life have singular value. It is not sufficient to pay lip-service: women play a central role in society, and policies and resources must reflect and recognize that they are not peripheral.

Women are not an optional extra, an item on the political agenda which comes and goes at the capricious whim of predominantly male politicians and policy-makers. They are here to stay, and they matter. Counsellors and therapists, if they are to avoid acting as agents of psychological sanctions which reinforce the patriarchal status quo, need to be aware of the various levels of women's experience. It is important that perspectives (such as the feminist position) which take account of the power and influence of structures, are not seen as intrinsically in conflict and competition with those which recognize the significance of individual history and dynamics. Locating the source of women's unhappiness and distress totally in the world outside them denies them their own individual validity. Similarly, identifying the source as simply coming from within them is isolating and alienating. Examining how these two may converge, blend and conflict is not straightforward, but neither are the lives of women.

This book has examined the interwoven strands that arise from history, family, political and societal structures, as well as from individual dynamics. At various points, I have alluded to myths that relate to or affect women: the returning hero in war time, when women were expected to retire quietly into domesticity; glorious motherhood, which fails to mention loss of independence and exhaustion; marriage as the great protector of women, when the person it protects is the man; men as protectors, when for many women they are the perpetrators of violence. The list is long – there are many more. Although it would be impossible to analyse all the myths about women at this point, there are some that appear with such monotonous regularity, that they need dismantling. Myths are powerful: it is easy to become seduced into accepting them. It is important that counsellors and therapists working with women extricate themselves from the mire of myths, and move onto firmer ground, where realities and fantasies are less inextricably mixed. These myths have some things in common. They attempt to devalue women. They distort and ridicule. They obliterate or disguise the true qualities which women have. They are negative and destructive. And, of course, they are maintained predominantly by men. The perpetuation of myths can be seen as an attempt to subjugate women, to deny and distort their attributes and skills, and to undermine their self-confidence and belief in what they can offer. Myths exist within the context of an implicit and basic assumption: that male behaviour is both correct and the ideal to which everyone, including women, should conform. Any deviation from male-prescribed norms is seen as unacceptable. In this way, deviations are not seen as arising from the challenge of a different perspective, which may lead to changes. They are viewed as coming from inferiority or lack of sufficient understanding.

So, what are the commonly held and expressed myths? And what might be the reality behind them?

'Women are too emotional'

This myth suggests that women respond to situations inappropriately and with too great a show of emotion. There is a strong inference here that men are calm and sensible and rely on common sense. Emotions are merely a female indulgence. The fantasy is of the strong man coping bravely with adversity, while supporting a weeping woman.

Turning the myth around, a different interpretation becomes available. In working with women it becomes clear that they are more in touch with feelings and better at coping with them – both in themselves and in others. Perhaps this is why men in distress are far more likely to turn to a woman for help and comfort than to a man. At the level of understanding what another person is feeling and experiencing, women are generally far more astute than men. Women are not scared by their emotions; they are able to locate, acknowledge, and express them, and to allow others to do the same. Perhaps if men were encouraged to do the same, they would become less destructive.

How might this myth operate in counselling and therapy? Both men and women, counsellors and clients, can become drawn in. I illustrated in Chapter 4 how a woman attempting to express anger became defined as hysterical and over-emotional. Her real and justified emotional response was thereby conveniently hidden and avoided, and its expression controlled and contained by all the men present. She was left feeling she had been utterly unreasonable. Another depressed client recalled her partner's response to her when she challenged him after an argument. She was feeling very hurt and rejected. He had unilaterally taken a major decision that had long-term repercussions. When she finally plucked up courage to tackle him on this, he told her that she was being a 'typical woman', making a fuss about nothing; that she was immature, and did not know when she was well off. In this way he avoided all responsibility for his own actions. He got away with a somewhat immature response, in the guise of being the competent man. It is therefore important that in counselling women are assured that they have a right to their own feelings.

'Women are the weaker sex'

This myth can refer to physical strength and ability; it can justify the exclusion of women from certain jobs and careers; and it implies more generally that women are simply less able to cope.

The experience of women in the two world wars has demonstrated their ability to cope with an enormous range of jobs previously designated for men only. But women have always carried out heavy tasks, such as carrying children and shopping, and pushing laden prams, which require considerable energy, strength and stamina. For earlier generations housework was especially arduous and heavy.

Women have this stamina and strength, and they often cope with a long working day, as well as with the demands of their children (and men). But they not only show physical stamina; they also constantly demonstrate their psychological flexibility as they adjust rapidly from one set of demands to another, responding appropriately to each.

Childbirth and childcare are similarly demanding. To counter the myth of women as the weaker sex, we only need to consider a few basic facts: fewer girl babies than boy babies die in the first few weeks following birth; women live longer than men, and (as I pointed out in Chapter 6) in terms of their mental health they are more successful at living alone. This in no way substantiates the picture of 'the weaker sex'. What the myth does is to provide a convenient rationalization for discriminatory practices against women. Being labelled as 'weaker' from an early age has a powerful effect. It is easy for girls, especially as they enter adolescence but also in adulthood, to conform to this myth, for fear otherwise of being seen as lacking in femininity and, therefore, acceptability:

> Few men like to compete with, or be beaten by a woman. Since her status is inferior, it reflects badly on the men beneath her. There are areas in which girls and women can succeed, indeed excel, but these are the ones in which few men even bother to compete.[1]

Counselling can assist a woman in identifying her own strengths while also acknowledging her vulnerabilities. It is important to recognize that to identify the existence of one does not invalidate acknowledging the reality of the other. Myths oversimplify. Counselling and therapy can provide a counterbalance to them by recognizing contradictions, conflicts and ambivalences. In doing this, the counsellor can travel with her client along the road to more complete autonomy. At some point, of course, the client has to travel on alone, but at the start she often feels she has few strengths. In fact she has many, although perhaps not in a male-defined way: 'But when women start to perceive forms of strength based on their own life experiences, rather than believing they should have the qualities they attribute to men, they often find new definitions of strength.'[2]

But discovering these can be frightening, too. To do so is to challenge the myth. That can seem a dangerous position to be in, and one which women have not been prepared for. A client expressed this feeling:

> When I first came to see you I think I was like a little girl: frightened, cross, and unable to do anything. I think I've got to the stage of leaving home now. I've got to be grown up now. I haven't got any excuses any more. I am able to make my own decisions, and lead my own life. I am responsible in some ways, in some areas of my life, if anything goes wrong. It is exciting, but sometimes I don't like that.

'Women talk too much'

If we turn this myth on its head, it is more valid to argue that girls and women are better communicators than men. Being with a group of women, it is impressive to see how rapidly they communicate with one another, and the ease with which they share quite intimate information. They are also able to listen and create an atmosphere that is conducive to safety and confidence-sharing.

My own observations, shared with many others, are that women in mixed gender groups say far less than the men. Women freely and fluently communicate in single-sex groups, but they are inhibited by the presence of men. My experience of teaching mixed-gender groups of adults, even when there are fewer men, is that men interrupt more and take a disproportionate amount of the time. This is borne out by research findings relating to both adults and children:

> In classroom discussion boys predominated: for every four boys who participated, there was only one girl. When teachers asked questions they asked two boys to every one girl, and when teachers provided praise and encouragement three boys received it to every one girl. And in these classes there were more girls than boys.[3]

Studies of adult behaviour in small, mixed-gender groups produce similar findings[4]. Men talk more; they initiate more conversations, and they interrupt conversations more frequently than women. As another study points out, 'if women limit how much they talk in small groups, particularly work groups, they are less likely to be cast in leadership roles'.[5] In this way, a quality and ability which women clearly possess, that of effective verbal communication, is repressed. When women are with men, they worry that they will reinforce or confirm the myth. So they lose out. It seems they cannot win either way.

'Women are illogical'

An immediate retort to this is that it is men who are rigid in their thinking. They are trained to think in straight lines, rather than to be exploratory and flexible. They expect to find answers, and they have developed an academic model of learning and problem resolution that is male-orientated and male-dominated. It assumes that it is the only model, and that it is intrinsically correct rather than intrinsically biased. Yet this model has no room for, no awareness of or interest in the possibility of there being gender differences in thinking. Something which may seem logical to a man, can seem like crass stupidity or a gross oversimplification to a woman. Of course, men can say that women are intuitive, but this is based on subjectivity and therefore invalid. But it should not be automatically assumed that either the male or the female assessment of the other is superior or more correct. Despite this obvious truth, the assumption persists that the male view is correct, and that women have somehow got it wrong.

It should be remembered that higher education in the UK is dominated by men: there are very few women academics, and the higher up the professional ladder, the smaller their number. Throughout history men have dominated academic institutions. The theories they have developed have come from the male world of which they are a part. Even when their theories were fairly obviously mistaken, and indeed later proved to be false, they carried with them the stamp of male authority.

Women clients often express anxieties about 'being silly', 'not making sense' or being 'stupid'. They find it hard to trust their own judgement, or to recognize that their way of making sense of things is not invalid just because it differs from a male view. Women, if they are allowed to do so, are skilled at making connections, and following less obvious paths of thinking, which lead to new insights and perspectives. They are not illogical. They have a different way of approaching a problem or difficulty, whether it is an academic or a personal one.

'Women are bossy, and they nag'

It is very difficult for women to be heard, and it is hard for them to be assertive. Men who firmly state their point of view, and who are effective as organizers, are defined very differently from women who exhibit the same characteristics. Additionally, men are more fortunate in another respect: they are more likely to have been heard and noticed at the first time of speaking. Women are more likely to have been ignored, and either have to give in, or repeat what they have said.

Women who persist in stating their case until they have been heard invite a repertoire of demoralizing and diminishing responses. Whereas men can be assertive, powerful, determined, strong women are often described as being 'bossy', 'nagging', 'making a fuss', and 'being difficult'. Small wonder that many women who come for counselling find it difficult to assert themselves, either in their outside world or even in their counselling session.

One method some women have of avoiding the bossy or nagging label is to conform to the stereotype which is applied to women that to be feminine is to be pleasantly passive. Yet there is frequently a hidden agenda beneath the smiling and agreeable, façade. Inevitably, if this is discovered or emerges it can result in yet another label being applied – that of the 'manipulative' woman. The 'smiling through everything' presentation is one that will be familiar to those who work with women. It can cover unhappiness, fear and depression. Some women find it hard to let their counsellor see what lies behind the façade of compliance. They have been the recipients of too many messages for too long, telling them that to be acceptable to men they must conform to these myths.

Patriarchy, with its male power base, combines with the abundance of myths and stereotypes to create a situation in which women's visibility is obscured. They become shadowy figures, nearly always in the background, holding up male edifices. Without them, many of these would collapse. With them, male insecurities can be protected from public gaze and male acknowledgment. Both men and women lose out in this system. But female losses are inevitably greater. The system does not give them easy access to the power bases which would enable them to bring about changes in their lives. Counselling and psychotherapy can assist women in their attempts to make sense of the difficulties they experience. In this way women begin to experience themselves as people of substance, rather than shadows that merge with the background, changing shape and form to suit the order of the day. Women have become more visible. Counselling and therapy can facilitate this process, by encouraging them to give expression to their true experiences and their real feelings, and by actively acknowledging the validity of those experiences. Working with women in this way is valuable and valid not only for clients but also for their counsellors and therapists. It is an enriching and enlightening process to share. Women, as they move out of the darkness and into the light, may go through agonies and despair, but they also bring with them a warmth and an energy the light from which will not fade away.

Notes

1 Sharpe, S. (1976). *'Just Like a Girl.'* Penguin, p. 136.
2 Miller, J. Baker (1978). *Towards a New Psychology of Women.* Penguin, p. 38.
3 Spender, D. (1989). *Invisible Women.* The Women's Press, p. 55.

4 Lockheed, M.E. and Hall, K.P. (1976). 'Conceptualising sex as a status characteristic: Applications to leadership training strategies', *Journal of Social Issues* 32, 2, pp. 111–23.
5 Lipman-Blumen, J. (1984). *Gender Roles and Power*. Englewood Cliffs, NJ.: Prentice-Hall, p. 91.

Bibliography

Andrews, B. (1987). 'Violence in normal families', paper presented at Marriage Research Centre Conference on Family Violence, London, April.

Antonis, B. (1981). 'Mothering and motherhood', in Cambridge Women's Studies Group (eds), *Women in Society: Interdisciplinary Essays*. London: Virago Press.

Arieti, S. and Bemporad, J. (1978). *Severe and Mild Depression: the Psychotherapeutic Approach*. New York: Basic Books.

Auden, W.H. (1970). *A Certain World*. London: Faber and Faber.

Bachrach, L. (1975). 'Marital status and mental disorder', *Analytic Review Publication*, 75–217, Washington, DC: Dept. of Health, Education and Welfare.

Baran, G. (1987). 'Teaching girls science', in McNeil, M. (ed.) *Gender and Expertise*. London: Free Association Books.

Berger, J. (1972). *Ways of Seeing*. Harmondsworth: Penguin Books.

Berke, J. (1979). *I Haven't Had to Go Mad Here*. Harmondsworth: Penguin Books.

Berke, J. and Barnes, M. (1973). *Mary Barnes: Two Accounts of a Journey Through Madness*. Harmondsworth: Penguin Books.

Binney, V. (1981). 'Domestic violence: battered women in Britain in the 1970s', in Cambridge Women's Studies Group (eds), *Women in Society: Interdisciplinary Essays*. London: Virago Press.

Bowker, L. (1983). *Beating Wife Beating*. Lexington, Mass.: Lexington Books.

Bowlby, J. (1947). *Child Care and the Growth of Love*. Harmondsworth: Penguin Books.

Broverman, I., Broverman, D., Clarkson, F., Rosencrantz, P. and Vogel, S. (1970). 'Sex role stereotypes and clinical judgements of mental health', *Journal of Consulting and Clinical Psychology*, **34** (1), 1–7.

Brown, G. and Harris, T. (1978). *Social Origins of Depression*. London: Tavistock.

Bruch, H. (1984). *Eating Disorders: Obesity, Anorexia Nervosa and the Person Within*. London: Routledge and Kegan Paul.

Chaplin, J. (1988). *Feminist Counselling in Action*. London: Sage Publications.

Chesler, P. (1972). *Women and Madness*. New York: Doubleday.

Chodorow, N. (1978). *The Reproduction of Mothering*. London: University of California Press.

Cooper, C. (1971). *The Death of the Family*. Harmondsworth: Penguin Books.

Courtney, A. and Whipple, T. (1980). *Sex Stereotyping in Advertising*. Lexington, Mass.: Lexington Books.

Dahlberg, C. (1970). 'Sexual contact between patient and therapist', *Contemporary Psychoanalysis*, **6**, 107–24.

Dana, M. (1987). 'Abortion – a woman's right to feel', in Ernst, S. and Maguire, M. (eds), *Living with the Sphinx*. London: Women's Press.

Dana, M. and Lawrence, M. (1988). *Women's Secret Disorder: a New Understanding of Anorexia*. London: Grafton Books.

Davidson, V. (1981). 'Psychiatry's problem with no name: therapist-patient sex', in Howell, E. and Bayes, M. (eds), *Women and Mental Health*. New York: Basic Books.

DeFrancis, V. (ed.) (1967). *Sexual Abuse of Children*. Denver, Col.: American Humane Association.

Dinnerstein, D. (1987). *The Rocking of the Cradle and the Ruling of the World*. London: Women's Press.

Dobash, R.E. and Dobash, R.P. (1981). 'Community response to violence against wives: charivari, abstract justice and patriarchy', *Social Problems*, **28** (5), 563–81.

Dunbar, M. (1986). *Catherine: the Story of a Young Girl Who Died of Anorexia*. London: Viking.

Eichenbaum, L. and Orbach, S. (1983). *What Do Women Want?* London: Michael Joseph.

Eichenbaum, L. and Orbach, S. (1985). *Understanding Women*. Harmondsworth: Penguin Books.

Epstein, G. and Bronzaft, A. (1972). 'Female freshmen view their roles as women', *Journal of Marriage and the Family*, **34**.

The Equal Opportunities Commission. (1987). *Women and Men in Britain: A Statistical Profile*. London: HMSO.

The Equal Opportunities Commission. (1988). *Women and Men in Britain: A Research Profile*. London: HMSO.

Frazier, N. and Sadker, M. (1973). *Sexism in School and Society*. New York: Harper and Row.

Friedman, R.C. (ed.) (1982). *Behavior and the Menstrual Cycle*. New York: Marcel Dekker.

Garfinkel, P.E. 'The heterogeneity of anorexia nervosa-bulimia as a distinct sub-group', *Archives of General Psychiatry*, **37**, 1036–40.

Gayford, J. (1978). 'Battered wives', in Martin, J.P. (ed.), *Violence in the Family*. Chichester: John Wiley.

Goffman, E. (1961). *Asylums*. Harmondsworth: Penguin Books.

Goffman, E. (1963). *Stigma*. Englewood Cliffs, NJ: Prentice-Hall.

Gove, W.R. (1972). 'The relationship between sex roles, marital status and mental illness', *Social Forces*, **51**, 34–44.

Gove, W.R. and Tudor, F.J. (1973). 'Sex, marital status, and morality', *American Journal of Sociology*, **79**, 45–67.

Goz, R. (1981). 'Women patients and women therapists: some issues that come up in psychotherapy', in Howell, E. and Bayes, M. (eds), *Women and Mental Health*. New York: Basic Books.

Grabucker, M. (1988). *There's a Good Girl*. London: Women's Press.

Hanma, J. and Saunders, S. (1984). *Well-Founded Fear: a Community Study of Violence to Women*. London: Hutchinson.

Hartley, R. (1966). 'A developmental view of female sex-role identification', in Biddle, J. and Thomas, E.J. (eds), *Role Theory*. Chichester: John Wiley.

Hartup, W. (1963). 'Avoidance of inappropriate sex typing by young children', *Journal of Consulting Psychology*, **27**.

Henwood, M., Rimmer, L. and Wicks, M. (1987). *Inside the Family: Changing Roles of Men and Women*. London: Family Policy Studies Centre.

Heron, L. (1986). *Changes of Heart: Reflections on Women's Independence*. London: Pandora Press.

Hey, V. (ed.) (1989). *Hidden Loss: Miscarriage and Ectopic Pregnancy*. London: Women's Press.

Holmstrom, L. and Burgess, A. (1974). *Rape: Victims of Crisis*. Bowie, Md.: Brady.

Howell, E. (1981). 'Where do we go from here?', in Howell, E. and Bayes, M. (eds), *Women and Mental Health*. New York: Basic Books.

Howell, E. and Bayes, M. (eds). (1981). *Women and Mental Health*. New York: Basic Books.

Itzin, C. (1980). *Splitting Up*. London: Virago Press.

Kempe, H. (1962). 'The battered child syndrome', *Journal of the American Medical Association*, **181** (1), 17–22.

Kitzinger, S. (1975). 'The fourth trimester', *Midwife, Health Visitor and Community Nurse*, **11**, 118–21.

Laing, R. and Esterson, A. (1964). *Sanity, Madness, and the Family*. London: Tavistock.

Lee, C. (1983). *The Ostrich Position*. London: Writers and Readers Co-op.

Lipman-Blumen, J. (1984). *Gender Roles and Power*. Englewood Cliffs, NJ: Prentice-Hall.

Loban, G. (1976). *Sex Roles in Reading Schemes*. Children's Rights Workshop.

Lockheed, M.E. and Hall, K.P. (1976). 'Conceptualising sex as a status characteristic: applications to leadership training strategies', *Journal of Social Issues*, **32** (2), 111–23.

Lovell, A. 'When a baby dies', *New Society*, 4 August 1983.

MacLeod, S. (1981). *The Art of Starvation*. London: Virago Press.

Martin, D. (1976). *Battered Wives*. San Francisco: Glide Publications.

Masters, W.H. and Johnson, V.E. (1970). *Human Sexual Inadequacy*. Boston: Little Brown.

Melville, J. (1984). *The Tranquilliser Trap*. Glasgow: Fontana.

Miller, A. (1984). *Thou Shalt Not Be Aware*. London: Pluto Press.

Miller, J. Baker (1978). *Towards a New Psychology of Women*. Harmondsworth: Penguin Books.

Ministry of Education. Central Advisory Council for Education (England) (1963). *Half Our Future*. (Newsom Report). London: HMSO.

Minuchin, S. (1978). *Psychosomatic Families: Anorexia in Context*. Cambridge Mass.: Harvard University Press.

Mitchell, J. (1975). *Psychoanalysis and Feminism*. Harmondsworth: Penguin Books.

Mitchell, J. (1971). *Woman's Estate*. Harmondsworth: Penguin Books.

Monahan, L. *et al.* (1974). 'Intraphysic versus cultural explanations of the fear of success motives', *Journal of Personality and Social Psychology*, 29.

Moss, H.A. (1967). 'Sex, age, and state as determinants of mother-infant interaction', *Merrill Palmer Quarterly*, 13, 19–36.

Moss, P. (1988). Consolidated Report to the European Commission.

Neustatter, A. and Newson, G. (1986). *Mixed Feelings: The Experience of Abortion*. London: Pluto Press.

Newson, E. and Newson, J. (1976). *Seven Years Old in the Home Environment*. London: George Allen & Unwin.

Oakley, A. (1979). *Becoming a Mother*. Oxford: Martin Robertson.

Orbach, S. (1986). *Hunger Strike*. London: Faber and Faber.

Orbach, S. and Eichenbaum, L. (1987). 'Separation and intimacy', in Ernst, S. and Maguire, M. (eds), *Living with the Sphinx*. London: Women's Press.

Owen, U. (ed.) (1983). *Fathers: Reflections by Daughters*. London: Virago Press.

Pahl, J. (ed.) (1985). *Private Violence and Public Policy*. London: Routledge and Kegan Paul.

Palazzoli, M.S. (1974). *Self-Starvation: From the Intrapsychic to the Transpersonal Approach to Anorexia Nervosa*. London: Human Context Books.

Perry, J.A. (1976). 'Physicians' erotic and non-erotic physical involvement with patients', *American Journal of Psychiatry*, 133, 838–40.

Pizzey, E. and Shapiro, J. (1982). *Prone to Violence*. London: Hamlyn.

Rawlings, E. and Carter, D. (1977). 'Feminist and non-sexist psychotherapy', in Rawlings, E. and Carter, D. (eds), *Psychotherapy for Women*. Springfield, Illinois: Charles C. Thomas.

Richman, N. (1976). 'Depression in mothers of preschool children', *Journal of Child Psychology and Psychiatry*, 17, 75–8.

Reid, R.L. and Yen, S.S.C. (1981). 'Premenstrual syndrome', *American Journal of Obstetric Gynaecology*, 139 (1), 85–104.

Rohrbaugh, J.B. (1981). *Women: Psychology's Puzzle*. London: Sphere Books.

Sarsby, J. (1983). *Romantic Love and Security*. Harmondsworth: Penguin Books.

Seiden, A. (1976). 'Overview: Research on the psychology of women.

Women in families, work, and psychotherapy', *American Journal of Psychiatry*, **133**.

Sharpe, S. (1976). *'Just Like a Girl'*. Harmondsworth: Penguin Books.

Sharpe, S. (1984). *Double Identity: the Lives of Working Mothers*. Harmondsworth: Penguin Books.

Showalter, E. (1987). *The Female Malady: Women, Madness, and English Culture 1830–1980*. London: Virago Press.

Smith, L. (1989). *Domestic Violence: an Overview of the Literature*. London: HMSO.

Spender, D. (1989). *Invisible Women*. London: Women's Press.

Stricker, J. (1977). 'Implications of research for psychotherapeutic treatment of women', *American Psychologist*, **32**.

Tennov, D. (1976). *Psychotherapy: The Hazardous Cure*. New York: Anchor Press/Doubleday.

Winnicott, D.W. (1971). *Playing and Reality*. London: Tavistock.

Wolf, T. (1973). 'Effects of live modelled sex-inappropriate behaviour in a naturalistic setting', *Developmental Psychology*, **9**.

Woolley, P.V. and Evans, W.A. (1955). 'The significance of skeletal lesions in infants resembling those of traumatic origin', *Journal of the American Medical Association*, **158** (7), 539–43.

Worrell, J. (1981). 'New directions in counselling women', in Howell, E. and Bayes, M. (eds), *Women and Mental Health*. New York: Basic Books.

Index